中医药文化认同与传播（双语版）

The Cultural Recognition and Communication of Traditional Chinese Medicine

主编　井晓磊　尹　丽

Chief Editors Jing Xiaolei Yin Li

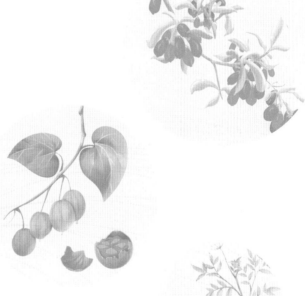

郑州大学出版社

图书在版编目（CIP）数据

中医药文化认同与传播 = The Cultural Recognition and Communication of Traditional Chinese Medicine：汉英对照／井晓磊，尹丽主编. -- 郑州：郑州大学出版社，2023. 12
ISBN 978-7-5645-9922-5

Ⅰ. ①中…　Ⅱ. ①井…②尹…　Ⅲ. ①中国医药学-文化-研究-汉、英　Ⅳ. ①R2-05

中国国家版本馆 CIP 数据核字（2023）第 180768 号

中医药文化认同与传播
ZHONGYIYAO WENHUA RENTONG YU CHUANBO

策划编辑	薛晗		封面设计	曾耀东
责任编辑	薛晗		版式设计	曾耀东
责任校对	张彦勤		责任监制	李瑞卿

出版发行	郑州大学出版社		地　址	郑州市大学路 40 号（450052）
出 版 人	孙保营		网　址	http://www.zzup.cn
经　销	全国新华书店		发行电话	0371-66966070
印　刷	河南文华印务有限公司			
开　本	787 mm×1 092 mm　1／16		彩　页	4
印　张	13.5		字　数	338 千字
版　次	2023 年 12 月第 1 版		印　次	2023 年 12 月第 1 次印刷

书　号	ISBN 978-7-5645-9922-5		定　价	59.00 元

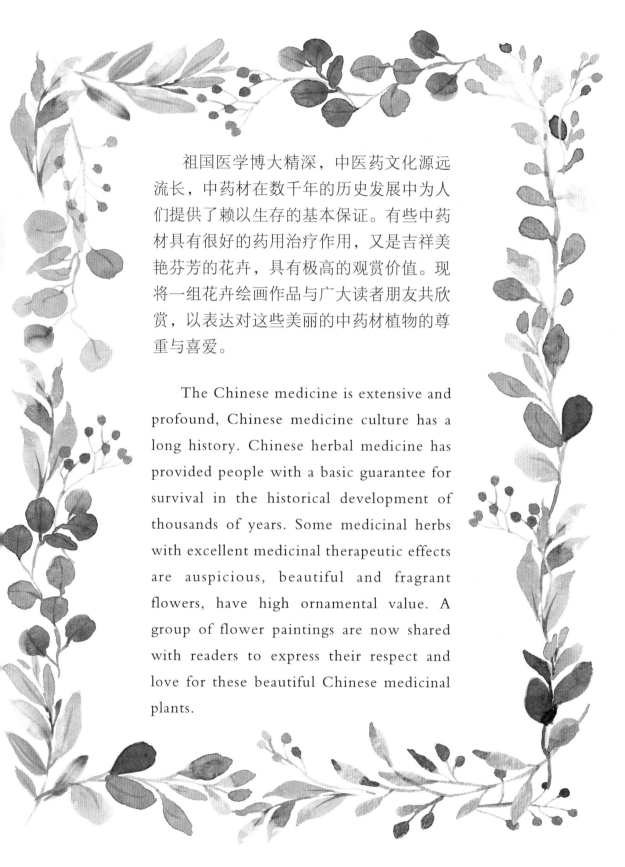

　　祖国医学博大精深，中医药文化源远流长，中药材在数千年的历史发展中为人们提供了赖以生存的基本保证。有些中药材具有很好的药用治疗作用，又是吉祥美艳芬芳的花卉，具有极高的观赏价值。现将一组花卉绘画作品与广大读者朋友共欣赏，以表达对这些美丽的中药材植物的尊重与喜爱。

　　The Chinese medicine is extensive and profound, Chinese medicine culture has a long history. Chinese herbal medicine has provided people with a basic guarantee for survival in the historical development of thousands of years. Some medicinal herbs with excellent medicinal therapeutic effects are auspicious, beautiful and fragrant flowers, have high ornamental value. A group of flower paintings are now shared with readers to express their respect and love for these beautiful Chinese medicinal plants.

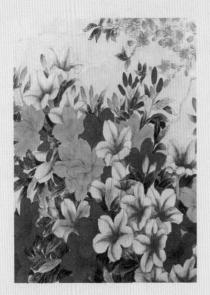

杜鹃花：祛湿调血、镇咳平喘

Rhododendron: Dispelling dampness and regulating blood, suppressing cough and relieving asthma

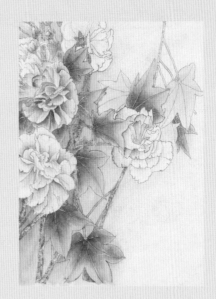

蜀葵：和血润燥、通利二便

Althaea rosa: Harmonizing blood and moistening dryness, promoting stool and urine

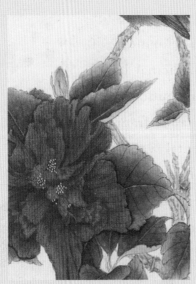

扶桑：清热解毒、凉血止血

Fusang (hibiscus rosa-sinensis): Clearing heat and removing toxin, cooling blood and stopping bleeding

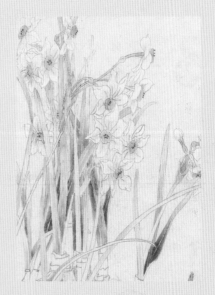

水仙：清热解毒、解郁散结

Narcissus: Clearing heat and removing toxin, releasing depression and dissipating bind

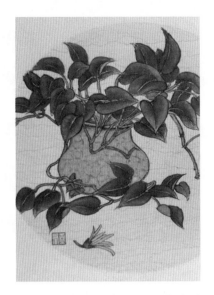

绿萝：降低血糖、抗菌消炎

Greens: Lowering blood sugar, antibacterial and anti-inflammatory

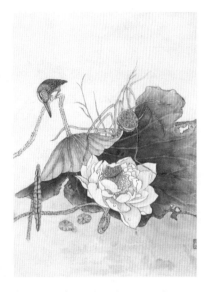

荷花：清热解暑、调节血脂

Lotus: Dispelling summer-heat and clearing heat, regulating blood lipids

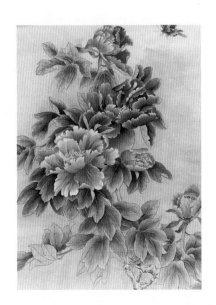

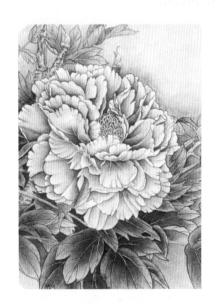

牡丹：清热凉血、活血化瘀

Peony: Clearing heat and cooling blood, activating blood circulation to dissipate blood stasis

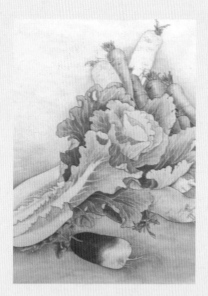

白菜、萝卜：清热化痰、促进消化

Chinese cabbage and radish: Clearing heat and resolving phlegm, promoting digestion

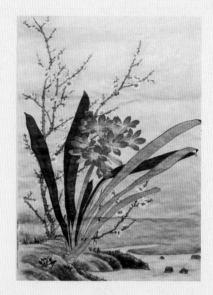

朱顶红：活血解毒、散瘀消肿

Hippeastrum: Activating blood to remove toxin, breaking stasis and dispersing swelling

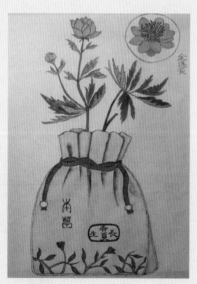

金莲花：清热解毒、消肿明目

Nasturtium: Clearing heat and removing toxin, resolving swelling and improving vision

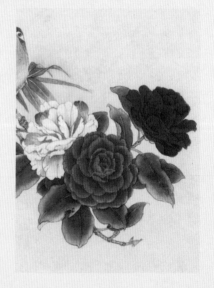

山茶花：凉血止血、散瘀消肿

Camellia: Cooling the blood and stopping bleeding, breaking stasis and dispersing swelling

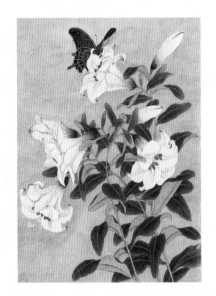

百合花：养阴清热、养颜美容

Lily: Nourishing *yin* and clearing heat, beautifying the skin

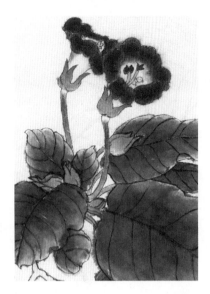

岩桐：利湿消肿、清热解毒

Yantong (Sinningia): Draining dampness and resolve swelling, clearing heat and removing toxin

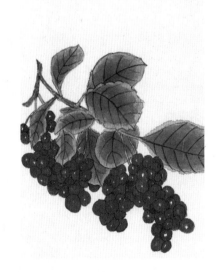

五味子：补肾安神、敛肺滋肾

Schisandra chinensis: Tonifying the kidney and tranquilizing spirit, astringing the lung and nourishing the kidney

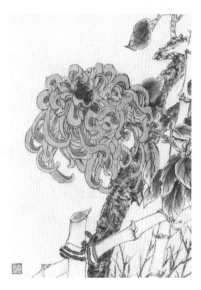

菊花：降血压、明目提神

Chrysanthemum: Lowering blood pressure, improving vision and refreshing the mind

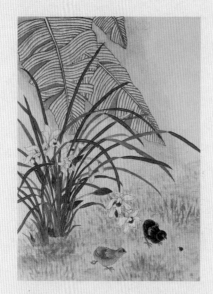

兰花：滋养阴液、生津润喉

Orchid: Nourishing *yin* fluids, promoting body fluids and moistening the throat

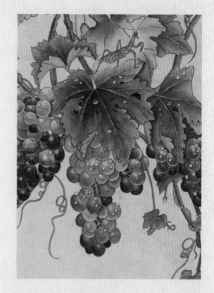

葡萄：生津消食、补血益气

Grape: Promoting body fluids and resolving food stagnation, tonifying blood and benefiting *qi*

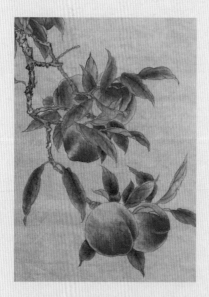

桃：生津润肠、美容养颜

Peach: Promoting body fluids and moistening the intestine, beautying the skin

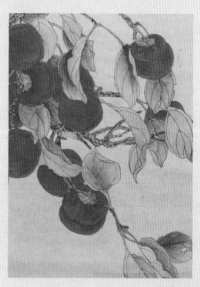

柿子：润肺生津、缓解便秘

Persimmon: Moistening the lung and promoting body fluids, relieving constipation

作者名单

主　编　井晓磊　尹　丽

副主编　刘玲霞

编　委　张世远　周一帆　赵丽莎　武亚琪

主　译　蒋宜轩

译　者　赵梅竹　杨盈盈

// Editorial Staff //

Chief Editors

 Jing Xiaolei Yin Li

Vice Chief Editor

 Liu Lingxia

Editorial Board Members

 Zhang Shiyuan Zhou Yifan Zhao Lisha Wu Yaqi

Chief Translator

 Jiang Yixuan

Translators

 Zhao Meizhu Yang Yingying

前　言

文化是一个国家与民族的灵魂，是铸牢中华民族共同体意识的根本精神依托和深厚的思想资源。中医药文化是中华优秀传统文化中不可或缺的重要组成部分，是中国文化软实力的重要标签。作为中华优秀传统文化的重要组成部分，中医药文化集中体现了中华民族的核心价值、思维方式。《中医药发展战略规划纲要(2016—2030年)》中指出，大力弘扬中医药文化，积极推动中医药国际发展是中医药发展战略的重要任务之一。

随着全球文化大融合的到来，中医药文化必须走出去，而提升中医药文化认同感是中医药文化走出去的重要保障。如何弘扬中医药文化、如何提高中医药文化自信、如何实现中医药文化国际化传播是当今中医药文化发展的时代主题。近代以来，我国在学习西方文明、反思东方文明的历史进程中，对西方现代医学的崇拜在客观上使中医药学遭遇到了前所未有的信任危机，被贴上了"非科学""过时"和"无用"等标签，集中体现中医药学本质与特色的中医药文化也因此颇受质疑，其传播和发展也陷入困境。面对这样的状况，我们必须从现实出发，积极提升中医药文化认同感和开展中医药文化国际化传播，有力回应中医药所遭受的一系列诘责，进而做到坚定中医药文化自信。

目前由于市面上适合海外人员阅读的外语版中医药著作较少，或者现存著作翻译水平参差不齐无法达到易读易懂，尤其是中医药文化内涵丰富但晦涩难懂，如"辨证论治""天人合一""阴阳学说""五行学说"等，对很多没有接触过中医药文化的海外人员来说势必难以理解。本书篇幅有限，因而精选部分章节进行翻译，尤其适用于初学者和外国留学生，是一本能满足其相应学习需求的汉英对照版著作。本书用通俗易懂的语言讲解博大精深的中医药概念,使更多的人认识、体会中医药文化的魅力与实力,架构文化传播桥梁,增强中医药文化的感召力和吸引力。

本书共有六篇,科学系统地阐述了中医药文化的历史起源和发展现状、中医药文化理论内涵,以期帮助人们认识了解中医药文化;详细介绍了中医日常保健技术以及中医养生与食疗知识,这是中医药文化在当今时代的创新性转化与发展,是中医药文化与现代健康理论相融相通的成果;最后总结了中医药文化认同现状、中医药文化国际传播中的机遇与挑战等,展示了中医药文化的独特魅力。

本书为河南省中医药文化与管理研究重点项目(TCM2022007)的主要研究成果之一。本书的出版,凝聚了编写团队的集体智慧与辛勤劳动,同时河南中医药大学第一附属医院退休教师、河南省美术家协会会员高亚君女士为本书手绘了精美插图,河南省卫生健康委员会给予了大力支持,在此一并致以衷心的感谢! 希望本书能对广大读者有所裨益。由于水平有限,不足之处,敬请各位读者提出宝贵意见,以便再版时修订提高!

编　者

2023 年 5 月

Preface

Culture, the soul of a country and a nation, is the fundamental spiritual support and profound ideological resource for building the consciousness of the Chinese nation community. Traditional Chinese medicine culture, an indispensable part of Chinese excellent traditional culture, is consideredas an important label of Chinese cultural soft power. As an important part of Chinese excellent traditional culture, Chinese medicine culture embodies the core values and thinking mode of the Chinese people. *The Outline of Strategic Planning for the Development of Traditional Chinese Medicine* (*2016 – 2030*) points out it is one of the important tasks of the development strategy of traditional Chinese medicine to vigorously carry forward the Chinese medicine culture and actively promote the international development of traditional Chinese medicine.

With the arrival of global culturalfusion, Chinese medicine culture must go out, soit is an important guarantee for Chinese medicine to go out for enhancing the sense of Chinese medicine cultureidentity. There are the themes of the times in the development of Chinese medicine culture, such as how to spread Chinese medicine culture, how to improve self-confidence of Chinese medicine culture and how to realize international dissemination of Chinese medicine culture. Since modern times, in the historical process of learning Western civilization and reflecting Eastern civilization, the worship of Western modern medicine objectively caused Chinese medicine to encounter an unprecedented crisis of trust, which was labeled as "unscientific", "outdated" and "useless". Therefore, Chinese medicine culture, which embodies the essence and characteristics of Chinese medicine, is questioned. Also its dissemination and development are also in trouble. Faced with such a situation, it must proceed from reality to actively enhance the sense of Chinese medicine culture identity, to carry out the international dissemination of Chinese medicine culture, to effectively respond to a series of responsibilities suffered by Chinese medicine. Finally, it will strengthen the confidence of Chinese medicine culture.

At present, there are few foreign language versions of Chinese medicine workssuitable for overseas people to read in the market, or the books' levelsvary dramatically in translation, which is not easy to read and understand. In particular, Chinese medicine culture is rich in content but difficult to understand, such as "syndrome differentiation and treatment", "harmony between man and nature", "yin-yang theory" and "five elements theory", which are so difficult for many overseas people who have not been exposedto the knowledge of traditional Chinese medicine. This book selecting the content of Chinese medicine culture communication, is especially suitable for beginners and foreign students. It is a Chinese-English bilingual book that can meet the corresponding learning needs. This book explains the profound concept of Chinese medicine in easy-to-understand language, so that more people can know and experience the charm and strength of Chinese medicine culture, build a bridge of cultural communication, and enhance the appeal and attraction of Chinese medicine culture.

There are six articles in this book, which scientifically and systematically expound the historical origin and development status of Chinese medicine culture and the theoretical connotation of Chinese medicine culture, in order to help people understand Chinese medicine culture; This paper introduces the daily health care technology of traditional Chinese medicine and the knowledge of keeping in good health and food therapy of traditional Chinese medicine, which is the innovative transformation and development of traditional Chinese medicine culture in the present era and the result of the integration of traditional Chinese medicine culture and modern health theory; At the same time, this book summarizes the current situation of Chinese medicine culture identity, opportunities and challenges in the international dissemination of Chinese medicine culture, and shows the unique charm of Chinese medicine culture.

This book is one of the main research results of the *Research Project of Traditional Chinese Medicine Culture and Management in Henan Province* (TCM2022007). The publication of this book embodies the collective wisdom and hard work of the writing team. I would like to thank Ms. Gao Yajun, a retired teacher of the *First Affiliated Hospital of Henan University of Traditional Chinese Medicine* and a member of *Henan Artists Association*, for creating exquisite illustrations for this book. Thanks to the strong support from *Health Commission of Henan Province*. I hope this book will be beneficial to the readers. Due to some shortcomings, experts, peers and readers can put forward valuable opinions to revise. We will improve when this book reprints!

Authors
May,2023

目 录

第一章

中医药文化认同
(Cultural Identity of Traditional Chinese Medicine)

中医药文化凝聚着中华民族几千年的劳动智慧,是我国特有的传统文化,推动着中医药事业的持续发展。文化认同是人们对于一种文化所产生的情感上的共鸣,它能够转化为行为上的认可,是个体的自我认知和自我概念的重要组成部分。文化认同与民族、宗教或任何具有独特文化的社会群体关系密切。中医药文化认同是人们对中医药文化中所凝结的文化价值和文化价值功能等的认知,并表现出来的积极心理和相应的行为倾向。因此,中医药文化认同是文化认同在中医药领域的具体化形式。

Traditional Chinese medicine culture, embodying the wisdom of the Chinese nation for thousands of years, is considered as a unique traditional culture in China, which promotes the sustainable development of the traditional Chinese medicine industry. Cultural identity is the emotional resonance of people for a culture. It can be transformed into the behavioral recognition as an important component of individual self-cognition and self-concept. Cultural identity is closely related to nationality, religion or any social group with unique culture. As a part of Chinese culture, cultural identity of Traditional Chinese Medicine is defined as people's understanding of the cultural values and functions, the positive psychology and corresponding behavioral tendencies. Therefore, Chinese medicine cultural identity is a concrete form of cultural identity in the field of Chinese medicine.

第一节　文化认同与中医药文化认同
(Cultural Identity and Cultural Identity of
Traditional Chinese Medicine)

文化认同(cultural identity)指一个人对于自身属于某个社会群体的认同感,与心理学密切相关,是一个人的自我概念与自我认知。其对象往往与不同国籍、民族、宗教、社会阶层、世代、定居地或任何类型具有其独特文化的社会群体有关。文化认同不仅是个人特征,同时也是具有相同的文化认同或教养的人所组成群体的特征,主要参考心理学研究中的认同态度心理结构,分为认知、情感、行为三大维度。

中医药是我国独具特色的医疗资源,而中医药文化正是在医学实践发展过程中总结的优秀中华传统文化。中医药文化认同是文化认同在中医药领域的具体化形式。中医药文化认同(cultural identity of TCM)是个体对中医药文化积极的认知、体验和行为的综合体,是指对中医药文化的接纳和认可的态度,包括中医药文化认知(cultural cognition of TCM,CCTCM)、中医药文化情感(cultural emotion of TCM,CETCM)及中医药文化行为(cultural behavior of TCM,CBTCM)。

一、文化、认同与文化认同(Culture,Identity and Cultural Identity)

著名英国学者泰勒(Edward B. Tylor)将文化定义为:"文化或文明,就其广泛的民族学意义来说,是包括全部的知识、信仰、艺术、道德、法律、风俗以及作为社会成员的人所掌握和接受的任何其他的才能和习惯的复合体。"这说明文化是复杂的。文化与人类社会的组织方式、生活方式相联系,除了已经物化的文化形式,文化的核心则由意识、精神、观念构成,由此形成了各种形态的文化,使人们具有一定的文化特性。第一,文化具有习得性。文化不是遗传的,是在社会互动中学习而来的,因此人能不断适应不同的社会和自然环境。第二,文化具有稳定性。文化一旦形成,便具有强大的稳定性。文化包括物化的民风民俗、文字和语言等具有象征性的符号及文化的核心:意识、精神等。人们的精神世界在相应文化中,会产生自我认同,会归于不同的文化群体,从而产生归属感。久而久之,个体在不同群体中产生的归属感就具有稳定性,从而延续下来。第三,文化具有多元性。随着社会经济的发展,当2种或者多种不同文化相遇时,首先要解决的就是认同问题,将文化与认同结合起来,也就形成了文化认同。

认同(identity)是个体心理上的趋同过程,是个体在特定文化社会环境中受该文化影响后的自我确认和归属。奥地利心理学家 Freud 最早提出"认同"这一概念。他将认同看作一个心理过程,是个人向另一个人或团体的价值、规范与面貌去模仿、内化并形成自己行为模式的过程,认同是个体与他人有情感联系的原初形式。美国学者埃里克森(Erik H. Erikson)深入探讨了认同和个体早年经验的关系,认为认同是"一种熟悉自身的感觉,一种知道个人未来目标的感觉,一种从他信赖的人们中获得所期待的认可的内在自信",认同无处不在,对人们的生活产生着巨大的影响。此外,亨廷顿(Samuel P. Huntington)认为:个人有认同,群体也有认同;绝大多数情况下,认同都是构建起来的概念;个人有多重身份,包括归属性的、地域性的、经济的、文化的、政治的、社会的及国别的;认同是自我界定,但又是自我与他人交往的产物。后续研究中也有多位学者分别从哲学、心理学、政治学以及社会学角度来讨论认同的概念,并认为认同是某一或某些社会成员在社会互动过程中,通过对自我与他者的区分,自认为或被认为属于某个特定社会群体的同一性和归属感。如在心理学方面,认同是一个用来表示主体性、归属感的概念,它是维系人格与社会及文化之间互动的内在力量。从社会学的角度来看,认同是个人或者群体通过与固有事物的互动,确定互相之间的关系的过程,是个人和群体通过与外界做参照而意识到自身的不同的态度和行为。总体而言,基于以往研究,认同应包含认识辨明、同意承认、共同参与,在微观层面上,认同是人类行为的心理动力源泉,它坚定了人们对自己的看法;在宏观层面,认同是个人意义的深层代码,它将个人与最一般层面的社会意义相联系。从类型上看,认同包括种族认同、民族认同、社会(群体)认同、自我认同、文化认同等多种类型,但核心是文化认同。因为在民族认同、社会认同和自我认同中都包含着文化认同的内容。认同所蕴含的身份或角色合法性,都离不开文化。身份、角色、合法性,都只能在一定的文化中才能具有意义。即使是与认同不可分割的自我概念,也是文化的产物。

文化认同最早出现在西方学者研究的心理学、哲学和社会学领域,其定义也有上千种,文化认同对个人、社会、民族和国家都有着巨大作用。对个人而言,文化是个体识别的重要标志之一,也是个体确定自我身份和意义边界的坐标,是个体寻求同类和融入群体的标准和依据。文化认同为核心所构成的个体心理与思想体系,引导着个人的价值观念和日常行为。对社会群体而言,文化认同是群体形成的核心要素之一,是群体特性的表现,是区别"我们"和"他们"的依据,具有增强群体凝聚力的功能。对于民族和国家而言,没有成员共同的文化认同,民族团结和谐就没有根基,国家稳定富强也就没有民心基础。对于中华民族而言,中国人的文化认同不仅仅是安身立命之本,也是实现中华民族伟大复兴中国梦的文化心理基础。

综上所述,文化认同是人们对于文化的倾向性共识与认可,人们使用相同的文化符号、秉承共同的文化理念、遵循共同的思维方式和行为规范、追求共同的文化理想是文化认同的依据。文化认同反映着人们对文化的认识和接受程度,因而文化认同是一个由表及里逐渐发展的内化过程。根据文化认同的程度可将其分为 3 个层次:一是文化认同的表现层,即对文化形式的认同;二是文化认同的保护层,即对文化规范的认同;三是文化认同的核心层,即对文化价值的认同。3 个层次相互影响和相互作用,构成了文化认同的体系。

二、文化认同的根源（Origin of Cultural Identity）

有人认为,文化认同作为一种现象,早已存在,文化认同往往是文化冲突后的结果。但文化认同作为一个问题受到人们的关注,则是伴随着现代性及其引发的文化危机而出现的,现代性昭示了文化认同的真正根源。现代性导致文化认同问题凸显的最根本原因在于以社会化大生产为标志的现代社会改变了传统社会原有的结构和运行机制,人们原有的生活方式和交往方式发生了重大改变,打乱了传统社会原有的认同模式和认同格局,引发了真正意义上的认同危机。现代性在促使社会转型的同时,还直接引发了空前的文化危机,使文化认同成为突出的时代课题。这种文化危机集中表现在:首先,现代性对传统的否定在一定意义上造成了文化断裂。传统是文化中最具特色、最重要、最普遍、最有生命力的内容,也是文化认同的重要载体,而现代性是在对传统、传统文化的批判和超越过程中确立起来的。在现代性建构的过程中,总要对传统和传统文化有所批判、有所否定。而这种否定又必然影响人们对民族文化传统、传统文化的认同,促使人们建立新的文化认同。其次,伴随现代性而来的强势文化扩张和文化霸权,造成了文化秩序破坏和文化生态的失衡。而文化认同问题的提出,是对文化霸权的抗争,也是对弱势文化生存权的维护、对文化多样性的呼唤。最后,现代性所形成的"以物的依赖性为中介的个人独立性",带来了社会与人自身的普遍物化,特别是文化对人的否定和扭曲。现代性的核心是市场化,现代性文化的实质则是文化的物化与技术化。这种以技术和物化为特征的文化,不仅无法有效解决文化认同问题,且易导致人们自我认同的困惑。在这个意义上,现代性的文化危机就是人与文化关系的危机,即文化认同的危机。

三、中医药文化认同的概念(Concept of Cultural Identity of Traditional Chinese Medicine)

文献检索显示,中医药文化认同最早由王东坡提出:中医药学只有按照自己的文化认同,沿着自身的文化体系去发展、去创新,才能融入主流医学的领域。经学者研究与发展,中医药文化认同已经成为探索中医药文化传播的重要工具。潘小毅等定义中医药文化认同为:有意识或无意识状态下向个人灌输的具有中医药文化属性的知识、信念、情感、行为、价值观等方面的个体感知。中医药文化认同的形成有助于个体学习与发展传统中医药文化和加大与提升中医药文化的建设力度。与此同时,中医药文化作为中国国粹瑰宝,更是以其最优秀、最独特、最本质的国家文化软实力向世界展示中国风采。因此,国际中医药文化认同感的提升将促进国际中医药文化氛围的塑造,扩大中医药文化的国际影响力,推动中医药学走向世界,为世界人民生命健康做出中国贡献。

四、中医药文化认同的根源(Origin of Traditional Chinese Medicine Cultural Identity)

由于文化认同内容的变化和文化的多元化,便出现了文化认同的危机,各种文化认同之间也存在着挑战和竞争。当中医药文化认同出现了危机时,会引起中国人去寻找个体的合理性与归属感,从而提高中医药文化认同。中医药文化认同危机形成有两方面因素,一是多元文化之间的冲突,这里主要指的是中西医文化冲突,二是在文化认同内容的变化中,产生的中医药文化断层。

（一）中西医文化冲突

文化冲突与文化认同的关系是相互联系、相互补充的。从逻辑上来看，文化冲突最主要的是人们在文化方面，对自我身份、自我认知的冲突，文化冲突引起的文化认同危机，也刺激个体去寻找自我的合理性和存在性，从而提高了对文化的认同。因此，文化冲突引起文化危机，落脚到文化认同。从现象看，文化冲突对文化认同的影响表现在两个方面——首先，在《文化认同与全球化》中提到，随着霸权政治经济的到来，从而产生了强势文化，会引起由个体的文化冲突导致的文化认同危机，使弱势文化的文化认同受到挑战。其次，现代文化的发展，是在传统文化的批判和继承中发展而来的，在这种文化冲突的过程中，又促进人们对新的文化的认同。

在众多文化冲突里面，最为突出的是中西文化的冲突。在当代的文化冲突中，中西文化冲突已经成为影响最大、最广的文化现象。在频繁的中西文化交流之前，中西方各自都有着独立发展的文化历史，有属于自己的文化体系，但是这两种体系的内容和结构有很大的差异，这种巨大的差异也就造成了不可回避的文化冲突，随着全球一体化的进程加快，两者频繁地产生冲突。

中西医文化的冲突是中西文化冲突的缩影，最具代表性。中医药文化认同感的强弱，对于中医药文化的存在和发展起着重要的作用。如果中医药文化认同高，则在这种文化冲突下，不仅能存在，还能找到自己的发展和社会定位，焕发新的生机。而文化冲突引发的中医药文化危机只是开始，以西医为代表的外来文化在引发中医药文化认同危机的同时，也激发了中国人寻找适合的文化，从而激发文化自尊和文化自信。在文化多元化和现代社会转型的背景下，因中西医文化冲突，从而引发了中医药文化认同危机。

（二）中医药文化断层

文化发展的连续性，是一个国家、一个民族的传统文化能够发展和延续的保证，但只重视文化的连续性，就会忽视现代社会发展要求的文化与传统文化之间的巨大差异。文化的非连续性则是现代文化在今天得到提升的关键，但如果只重视文化的非连续性，那么就会进入文化的虚无主义。这种文化发展的非连续性，就是文化断层。在现今变化剧烈的社会中，文化断层和连续性都值得研究，而相对于文化连续性来说，文化断层更值得重视。所有的文化都有断层的现象，是非连续发展的。文化断层是源于文化认同内容的改变，主要受外部力和内驱力的影响。一方面，由于社会的快速转型，人们受到外界社会变化的压力，迫使其改变原有的文化认同，而整合新的文化认同，以适应变化的环境。另一方面，因为群体间的吸引力不同，一些群体在社会中的资源、权利、地位上更有优势，在这样的情况下，人们更愿意去认同更有吸引力的群体，从而改变原有的认同。随着时间的流逝，人们不断地整合新的文化内容到自身的文化认同中，对于传统文化的认同则慢慢减少。

中医药文化断层是从鸦片战争开始受到了西方的科学霸权主义的影响,导致部分人认为,与西医思维不同的中医是不科学的,甚至表现出难以理解的民族虚无主义。现今,中国人接受了科学教育,掌握的大多是数理化等现代科学文化知识,在短时间内掌握具有浓厚古文化的中医是很难的,在中医教学方面也造成了中医药文化断层。因此营销人员或者中医师为了便于具有"西方思维"的消费者理解,也就按照了西方"科学"的方式来解释中医。若照此下去,中医药文化非但不能还原本身的样貌,还会退化甚至消亡。

综上所述,中西医文化冲突与中医药文化断层产生的中医药危机,是中医药文化认同的根源所在。两者的共同作用,对个体、对中医药文化认同都有消极的影响,也是我们必须经历的痛苦。在面临外来文化的冲击,传统文化遭到抵触和打击的当下,对中医药文化认同的研究势在必行。

五、中医药文化认同的作用(Influence of Cultural Identity of Traditional Chinese Medicine)

现有研究普遍认为,培养和增强公众对中医药文化的认同,是中医药事业能够持续健康发展的重要保障,"国人只有在文化上认同中医药,才能在实际行动中支持中医药发展,中医药才能获得更广阔的未来"。另一方面,研究认为中医药学所肩负的已不仅仅是医学的本职,同时,还承担着中国传统文化薪火传递的重责。增强中医药文化认同能够确保我国传统文化主权和安全,提升国家软实力以及扩大国家影响力,亦能为社会主义核心价值体系提供传统文化素材和支撑。有学者甚至从 4 个方面分析了如何通过中医药文化认同的培育推动我国文化领域统战工作的开展。总体上,目前研究普遍认可,并强调中医药文化认同在多领域中的积极作用。

Traditional Chinese medicine culture, embodying the wisdom of the Chinese nation for thousands of years, is considered as a unique traditional culture in China, which promotes the sustainable development of the traditional Chinese medicine. Cultural identity is the emotional resonance of people for a culture. It can be transformed into the behavioral recognition as an important component of individual self-cognition and self-concept. Cultural identity is closely related to nationality, religion or any social group with unique culture. Cultural identity of traditional Chinese medicine is defined as people's understanding of the cultural values and functions, the positive psychology and corresponding behavioral tendencies. Therefore, the cultural identity of traditional Chinese medicine is a concrete form of cultural identity in the field of traditional Chinese medicine.

1 Cultural Identity and Cultural Identity of Traditional Chinese Medicine

Cultural identity refers to people's sense of identity that he or she belongs to a certain social group, which is closely related to psychology. It represents people's self-concept and self-awareness. Its object is often related to different nationalities, ethnicities, religions, social classes, generations, places of settlement or any type of social group with its unique culture. Cultural identity is not only an individual characteristic, but also a characteristic of groups formed by people with the same cultural identity or upbringing. Cultural identity mainly refers to the psychological structure of identity attitude in psychological research, which is divided into three major dimensions: cognitive, affective, and behavioral.

Traditional Chinese medicine is a unique medical resource in China, and the culture of Chinese medicine is precisely the excellent traditional Chinese culture summarized in the development of medical practice. Therefore, the cultural identity of traditional Chinese medicine is a concrete form of cultural identity in the field of traditional Chinese medicine. Cultural identity of Traditional Chinese Medicine (TCM) is a synthesis of individual's positive cognition, experience and behavior towards TCM culture, including cultural cognition of TCM (CCTCM), cultural emotion of TCM (CCTCM), and cultural behavior of TCM (CBTCM).

1.1　Culture, Identity and Cultural Identity

Edward B. Tylor, a famous British scholar, defines culture as: "Culture or civilization, in its broad ethnological sense, is a complex that includes all the knowledge, beliefs, arts, morals, laws, customs, and any other talents and habits mastered and accepted by the people who are members of the society." This shows that culture is complicated. Culture is linked to the organization and lifestyle of human society, encompassing both the cultural form materialized and the core of culture. This is composed of consciousness, spirit, and concepts, forming various forms of culture, which in turn gives rise to certain cultural characteristics. First, culture is learned. Culture is not hereditary, but is learned through social interaction, which enables individuals to continuously adapt to different social and natural environments. Second, culture is stable. Once a culture is formed, it has strong stability. Culture includes symbolic symbols such as materialized folk customs, characters and languages, as well as the core of culture: consciousness and spirit. In the context of the cultural group, people will develop self-identification and cultural identity, which will contribute to a sense of belonging. Over time, the sense of belonging generated by individuals in different groups becomes stable and thus continues. Third, culture has diversity. With the development of social economy, when two or more different cultures meet, the first thing to be solved is the issue of identity. By combining culture and identity, we form a cultural identity.

Identity is the process of psychological convergence of individuals, which is the self-identification and belonging of individuals after being influenced by that culture in a specific cultural and social environment. Austrian psychologist Freud first proposed the concept of "identity". He regarded identity as a psychological process, a process in which individuals imitate, internalize and form their own behavioral patterns towards the values, norms and appearance of another person or group. It's the original form of emotional connection between individuals and others. Erik H. Erikson, an American scholar, delved into the relationship between identity and individual's early experience, arguing that identity is "a feeling of familiarity with oneself, a feeling of knowing one's future goals, and an inner confidence in obtaining the desired recognition from the people he trusts". Identity is ubiquitous and has great influence on peoplel's lives. In addition, Samuel P. Huntington argued that individuals have identity and groups have identity. In most cases, identity is a constructed concept. Individuals have multiple identities, including attributive, regional, economic, cultural, political, social and national. Identity is self-defining, but it is also the product of self-interacting with others. Several scholars in subsequent studies have also discussed the concept of identity from the perspectives of philosophy, psychology, politics and sociology. They believe that identity is the distinction between oneself and others in the social interaction between certain social members or certain social members. For example, in psychology, identity is a concept used to express subjectivity and a sense of belonging. It is an internal force that maintains the interaction between personality and society and culture. From a sociological point of view, identity is a process in which individuals or groups determine their relationships with each other through interaction with inherent things. It is a process in which individuals and groups are aware of their different attitudes and behaviors through reference to the outside world. Generally speaking, based on previous studies, identity should contain recognition identification, consent recognition and joint participation. At the micro level, identity is the source of psychological motivation for human behavior, and it strengthens peoplel's views on themselves; At the macro level, identity is the deep code of personal meaning, which links the individual to the most general level of social meaning. In terms of types, identity includes racial identity, national identity, social (group) identity, self-identity, cultural identity and other types, but the core is cultural identity. On the one hand, it is because cultural identity is included in national identity, social identity and self-identity. The identity or role legitimacy implied by identity cannot be separated from culture. Identity, role, and legitimacy can only have meaning in a certain culture. Even the self-concept, which is inseparable from identity, is a product of culture.

Cultural identity first appeared in the field of psychology, philosophy and sociology studied by western scholars, and there are thousands of definitions of it, and cultural identity has a great effect on individuals, societies, nations and countries. For individuals, culture is one of the important indicators of individual identification as well as the coordinate for individuals to determine their own identity and meaning boundaries, and it is the standard and basis for individuals to seek similarity and integrate into groups. The individual psychology and thought system constituted by the core of cultural identity guides the values and daily behavior of individuals. For social groups, cultural identity is one of the core elements of group formation, a manifestation of the group's identity, a basis for distinguishing between "us" and "them" and has the function of strengthening group cohesion. For the nation and the country, without the common cultural identity of its members, there is no foundation for national unity and harmony, and there is no basis for the stability and prosperity of the state. For the Chinese nation, the cultural identity of the Chinese people is not only the foundation for a secure life, but also the cultural and psychological foundation for realizing the Chinese dream of the great rejuvenation of the Chinese nation.

In conclusion, cultural identity is people's tendentious consensus and recognition of culture, and it is the basis of cultural identity that people use the same cultural symbols, uphold common cultural concepts, follow common ways of thinking and behavioral norms, and pursue common cultural ideals. Cultural identity reflects peoplel's cognition and acceptance of culture, and thus cultural identity is a process of internalization that gradually develops from the outside to the inside. According to the degree of cultural identity, it can be divided into three levels: first, the manifestation layer of cultural identity, i. e. , identification with cultural forms; second, the protection layer of cultural identity, i. e. , identification with cultural norms; and third, the core layer of cultural identity, i. e. , identification with cultural values. The three levels influence and interact with each other, constituting the system of cultural identity.

1.2　Origin of Cultural Identity

According to Cui Xinjian, as a phenomenon, cultural identity has existed for a long time, and cultural identity is often the result of cultural conflict. However, the attention paid to cultural identity as an issue came with modernity and the cultural crisis it triggered, which revealed the true origin of cultural identity. The most fundamental reason for the prominence of cultural identity problems caused by modernity is that the modern society marked by socialized mass production has changed the original structure and operation mechanism of the traditional society, and people's original way of life and ways of communication have undergone significant changes, which have disrupted the original identification mode and pattern of the traditional society, and triggered an identity crisis in the true sense of the word. Modernity, while prompting social transformation, has also directly triggered an unprecedented cultural crisis, making cultural identity a prominent issue of the times. This cultural crisis is centered on the following: firstly, the negation of tradition by modernity has caused a cultural rupture in a certain sense. Tradition is the most distinctive, important, universal and vital content in culture, and it is also an important carrier of cultural identity, while modernity is established in the process of criticizing and surpassing tradition and traditional culture. In the process of constructing modernity, there is always a need to criticize and deny tradition and traditional culture. This negation in turn inevitably affects people's identification with national cultural traditions and traditional culture, prompting them to establish a new cultural identity; secondly, the strong cultural expansion and cultural hegemony that accompanies modernity has caused the destruction of cultural order and the imbalance of cultural ecology. The issue of cultural identity is a struggle against cultural hegemony, the maintenance of the right to survival of vulnerable cultures, and the call for cultural diversity; Finally, the "individual independence" formed by modernity has brought about the general materialization of society and people themselves, especially the negation and distortion of culture to people. The core of modernity is marketization, and the essence of modern culture is the materialization and technologization of culture. This kind of culture characterized by technology and materialization not only fails to effectively solve the problem of cultural identity, but also easily leads to the confusion of people's self-identification. In this sense, the cultural crisis of modernity is a crisis in the relationship between human and culture, i. e. , a crisis of cultural identity.

1.3 Concept of Cultural Identity of Traditional Chinese Medicine

The cultural identity of traditional Chinese medicine was first proposed by Wang Dongpo: Only by developing and innovating along its own cultural system in accordance with its own cultural identity can traditional Chinese medicine be integrated into the mainstream medical field. Through the research and development of scholars, the identification of traditional Chinese medicine culture has become an important tool for exploring the spread of traditional Chinese medicine culture. Pan Xiaoyi and others define the identity of traditional Chinese medicine culture as the individual perception of knowledge, beliefs, emotions, behaviors, values with the attributes of traditional Chinese medicine culture instilled in individuals consciously or unconsciously. The formation of traditional Chinese medicine cultural identity helps individuals to learn and develop traditional Chinese medicine culture, to increase and enhance the construction of Chinese medicine culture. At the same time, traditional Chinese medicine culture, as a national treasure of China, shows the Chinese style to the world with its best, unique and most essential national cultural soft power. Therefore, the enhancement of international Chinese medicine cultural identity will promote the shaping of international Chinese medicine cultural atmosphere, expand the international influence of traditional

Chinese medicine culture, promote Chinese medicine to the world, and make Chinese contributions to the lives and health of people around the world.

1.4　Origin of Traditional Chinese Medicine Cultural Identity

The change of cultural identity content and the diversification of cultural identity bring about the crisis of cultural identity, and there are challenges and competition among various cultural identities. When there is a crisis in the cultural identity of traditional Chinese medicine, it will cause Chinese people to look for individual rationality and sense of belonging, so as to improve the cultural identity of traditional Chinese medicine. There are two aspects in the formation of the cultural identity crisis of Chinese medicine, one is the conflict between multiple cultures, which here mainly refers to the cultural conflict between Chinese and Western medicine, and the other is the cultural fault of Chinese medicine that arises from the change in the content of cultural identity.

（1）Conflict Between Chinese and Western Medicine Cultures

The relationship between cultural conflict and cultural identity is interconnected and complementary. Logically, cultural conflict is most of all peoplel's cultural aspects, the conflict of self – identity, self – knowledge, cultural conflict caused by cultural identity crisis, but also stimulate the individual to find self–reasonableness and existence, which improves the identity of culture. Therefore, cultural conflict give rise to cultural crisis and finally to cultural identity. From the phenomena, the impact of cultural conflict on cultural identity is manifested in two aspects: firstly, as mentioned in "*Cultural Identity and Globalization*", with the advent of hegemonic politics and economy, a strong culture will emerge, which will cause individual cultural conflicts, and then develop into a cultural identity crisis, which will challenge the cultural identity of weak cultures. Secondly, modern culture develops through the criticism and inheritance of traditional culture, and in the process of cultural conflict, it promotes people's new cultural identity.

Among the many studies on cultural conflict, the most prominent one is the conflict between Chinese and Western cultures. In the contemporary cultural conflict, the cultural conflict between China and the West has become the most influential and widespread cultural phenomenon. With the acceleration of the process of global integration, before the frequent cultural exchanges between China and the West, each has its own independently developed cultural history and has its own cultural system, the content and structure of these two systems can be very different. This huge difference also creates an inescapable cultural conflict, which is what causes the two to clash frequently. With the advancement of globalization, the two cultural systems with large differences often produce fierce struggles and confrontations.

The conflict between Chinese and Western medicine culture is the epitome of the conflict between Chinese and Western culture, and is the most representative. The strength of Chinese medicine cultural identity plays an important role in the existence and development of traditional Chinese medicine culture. If traditional Chinese medicine has a strong cultural identity, it can not only survive in the midst of cultural conflicts, but also thrive and find its own path of development and social direction, thus gaining a new vitality. The crisis of traditional Chinese medicine culture caused by cultural conflict is only the beginning. The foreign culture represented by western medicine has triggered the crisis of cultural identity of Chinese medicine, but also stimulated Chinese to find a suitable culture, thus stimulating cultural self-esteem and cultural self-confidence. In the context of cultural pluralism and the transformation of modern society, the conflict between Chinese and western medicine cultures has triggered a crisis of cultural identity crisis of traditional Chinese medicine.

(2)Cultural Fault of Traditional Chinese Medicine

The continuity of cultural development is a guarantee that the traditional culture of a country or a nation can develop and continue, but to emphasize only the continuity of culture is to ignore the great difference between the culture required by the development of modern society, and the traditional culture. Cultural discontinuity is the key to the promotion of modern culture today, but if only the cultural discontinuity is valued, we will enter the cultural nihilism. This discontinuity in cultural development is the cultural fault. In today's society of drastic changes, both cultural fault and continuity are worth studying, and cultural fault is more worthy of attention than cultural continuity. All cultures are faulted and discontinuous in their development. The cultural fault is originated from the change of the content of cultural identity, which is mainly external force and internal drive. On the one hand, due to the rapid transformation of society, people are subjected to the pressure of external social changes, forcing them to change their original cultural identity and integrate a new one to adapt to the changing environment. On the other hand, because of the different attractiveness of groups, some groups have more advantages in terms of resources, power, and status in the society, under such circumstances, people are more willing to identify themselves with the more attractive groups, and thus change their original identities. As time passes, people continue to integrate new cultural contents into their own cultural identity, while the identity of traditional culture slowly decreases.

The cultural fault of traditional Chinese medicine began with the Opium Wars. Influenced by western scientific hegemony, some people believe that Chinese medicine, which is different from western medical thinking, is unscientific, and even shows an incomprehensible national nihilism. Nowadays, Chinese people have received scientific education and mastered most of the modern scientific and cultural knowledge such as mathematics, physics and chemistry, and it is very difficult to master Chinese medicine with a strong ancient culture in a short time, and the teaching of Chinese medicine has created a cultural fault line in Chinese medicine. Therefore, in order to make consumers with "western thinking" understand, marketers or Chinese medicine practitioners also follow the western "scientific" way to explain traditional Chinese medicine. If this continues, the culture of traditional Chinese medicine will not only fail to restore its own appearance but will also degenerate or even die out.

To summarize, the crisis of traditional Chinese medicine produced by the cultural conflict between Chinese and western medicine and the cultural fault of Chinese medicine is the origin of the cultural identity of traditional Chinese medicine. The joint effect of the two causes individuals to have a negative impact on the cultural identity of traditional Chinese medicine, and it is also the pain we must experience. In the face of the impact of foreign culture, traditional culture is confronted with resistance and blow, so it is imperative to study the identification of traditional Chinese medicine culture.

1.5 Influence of Cultural Identity of Traditional Chinese Medicine

Current researches generally believe that fostering andstrengthening the publicl's recognition of the culture of traditional Chinese medicine is an important guarantee for the sustainable and healthy development of the cause of traditional Chinese medicine. "Chinese people can only support the development of traditional Chinese medicine in practical actions and achieve a broader future of traditional Chinese medicine." On the other hand, the research holds that what traditional Chinese medicine shoulders is not only the responsibility of medicine, but also the heavy responsibility of the transmission of Chinese traditional culture. Zhou Zheng further summarized that strengthening the cultural identity of traditional Chinese medicine can ensure the sovereignty and security of China's traditional culture, enhance national soft power, and expand national influence. It can also provide traditional cultural materials and support for the socialist core value system. Deng Cuirong even analyzes how the cultivation of TCM cultural identity can promote the united front work in China's cultural field from four aspects. In general, the current researches generally recognize and emphasize the positive role of TCM cultural identity in multiple fields.

第二节　中医药文化认同的相关政策
（Policies Relating to Cultural Identity of Traditional Chinese Medicine）

一、关于扶持和促进中医药事业发展的若干意见（Opinions on Supporting and Developing the Traditional Chinese Medicine Industry）

2009 年 4 月 21 日,为进一步扶持和促进中医药事业发展,落实医药卫生体制改革任务,中共中央、国务院关于扶持和促进中医药事业发展提出若干意见。

第一,充分认识扶持和促进中医药事业发展的重要性和紧迫性。随着健康观念变化和医学模式转变,中医药越来越显示出独特优势。中医药作为中华民族的瑰宝,蕴含着丰富的哲学思想和人文精神,是我国文化软实力的重要体现。扶持和促进中医药事业发展,对于深化医药卫生体制改革、提高人民群众健康水平、弘扬中华文化、促进经济发展和社会和谐,都具有十分重要的意义。第二,发展中医药事业的指导思想和基本原则。坚持以邓小平理论和"三个代表"重要思想为指导,全面贯彻落实科学发展观。遵循中医药发展规律,保持和发扬中医药特色优势。第三,发展中医医疗和预防保健服务。推动中医药进乡村、进社区、进家庭,充分发挥中医预防保健特色优势。第四,推进中医药继承与创新。支持中医药科技创新,推动中药新药和中医诊疗仪器、设备的研制开发。第五,加强中医药人才队伍建设。第六,提升中药产业发展水平,促进中药资源可持续发展。第七,加快民族医药发展。改善就医条件,满足民族医药服务需求。第八,繁荣发展中医药文化。开展中医药科学文化普及教育,加强中医药文化资源开发利用,打造中医药文化品牌。第九,推动中医药走向世界。积极参与相关国际组织开展的传统医药活动,进一步开展与外国政府间的中医药交流合作,加强中医药知识和文化对外宣传,促进国际传播。第十,完善中医药事业发展保障措施等意见。各级政府要逐步增加投入,重点支持开展中医药特色服务、公立中医医院基础设施建设、重点学科和重点专科建设以及中医药人才培养。

二、"十四五"中医药发展规划（The "14th Five-Year Plan" for the Development of Traditional Chinese Medicine）

2022 年 3 月 3 日,为贯彻落实中共中央、国务院关于中医药工作的决策部署,明确"十四五"时期中医药发展目标任务和重点措施,依据《中华人民共和国国民经济和社会发展第十四个五年规划和 2035 年远景目标纲要》,国务院办公厅制定出本规划。

"十四五"中医药发展规划提出了 10 个主要任务:第一,建设优质高效中医药服务体系,做强龙头中医医院,做实基层中医药服务网络。第二,提升中医药健康服务能力。彰显中医药在健康服务中的特色优势,提升疾病预防能力。实施中医药健康促进行动,推进中医治未病健康工程升级。提高中医药公共卫生应急和重症救治能力,完善中药应急物资保障供应机制,持续开展少数民族医药文献抢救整理工作。第三,建设高素质中医药人才队伍,完善落实西医学习中医制度,加强中西医结合学科建设,培育一批中西医结合多学科交叉创新团队。第四,建设高水平中医药传承保护与科技创新体系,建立中医药传统知识数据库、保护名录和保护制度。第五,推动中药产业高质量发展。加强中药资源保护与利用和道地药材生产管理,提升中药产业发展水平。第六,发展中医药健康服务业。推广太极拳、八段锦等中医药养生保健方法和中华传统体育项目,以保健食品、特殊医学用途配方食品、功能性化妆品、日化产品为重点,研发中医药健康产品。第七,推动中医药文化繁荣发展。加强中医药文化研究和传播,加强中医药科普专家队伍建设,推动中医医疗机构开展健康讲座等科普活动。第八,加快中医药开放发展。积极参与全球卫生健康治理,推进中医药参与新型冠状病毒感染等重大传染病防控国际合作,分享中医药防控疫情经验。第九,深化中医药领域改革。建立符合中医药特点的评价体系,健全现代医院管理制度。第十,强化中医药发展支撑保障。加强关键信息基础设施、数据应用服务的安全防护,增强自主可控技术应用。

三、中医药发展战略规划纲要(2016 — 2030 年)[Outline of the Strategic Plan for the Development of Traditional Chinese Medicine (2016–2030)]

中医药作为我国独特的卫生资源、潜力巨大的经济资源、具有原创优势的科技资源、优秀的文化资源和重要的生态资源,在经济社会发展中发挥着重要作用。随着我国新型工业化、信息化、城镇化、农业现代化深入发展,人口老龄化进程加快,健康服务业蓬勃发展,人民群众对中医药服务的需求越来越旺盛,迫切需要继承、发展、利用好中医药,充分发挥中医药在深化医药卫生体制改革中的作用,造福人类健康。2017 年 5 月 12 日,为明确未来十五年我国中医药发展方向和工作重点,促进中医药事业健康发展,国务院制定本规划纲要。

《中医药发展战略规划纲要(2016—2030 年)》的重点任务概括如下。

(一)切实提高中医医疗服务能力

1.完善覆盖城乡的中医医疗服务网络。加强中医医院康复科室建设,支持康复医院设置中医药科室,加强中医康复专业技术人员的配备。

2.提高中医药防病治病能力。推动建立融入中医药内容的社区健康管理模式,开展高危人群中医药健康干预。

3. 促进中西医结合。推进中西医资源整合、优势互补、协同创新。积极创造条件建设中西医结合医院。完善中西医结合人才培养政策措施,建立更加完善的西医学习中医制度。

4. 促进民族医药发展。鼓励民族地区各类医疗卫生机构设立民族医药科,鼓励社会力量举办民族医院和诊所。

5. 放宽中医药服务准入。鼓励社会力量举办连锁中医医疗机构,对社会资本举办只提供传统中医药服务的中医门诊部、诊所,医疗机构设置规划和区域卫生发展规划不作布局限制。

6. 推动"互联网+"中医医疗。利用移动互联网等信息技术提供在线预约诊疗、候诊提醒、划价缴费、诊疗报告查询、药品配送等便捷服务。

(二)大力发展中医养生保健服务

1. 加快中医养生保健服务体系建设。加强中医医院治未病科室建设,为群众提供中医健康咨询评估、干预调理、随访管理等治未病服务。

2. 提升中医养生保健服务能力。鼓励中医药机构充分利用生物、仿生、智能等现代科学技术,研发一批保健食品、保健用品和保健器械器材。

3. 发展中医药健康养老服务。推动中医药与养老融合发展,促进中医医疗资源进入养老机构、社区和居民家庭。

4. 发展中医药健康旅游服务,以中医药文化传播和体验为主题,融中医疗养、康复、养生、文化传播、商务会展、中药材科考与旅游于一体的中医药健康旅游。

(三)扎实推进中医药继承

1. 实施中医药传承工程,全面系统继承历代各家学术理论、流派及学说,全面系统继承当代名老中医药专家学术思想和临床诊疗经验,总结中医优势病种临床基本诊疗规律。

2. 加强中医药传统知识保护与技术挖掘。开展对中医药民间特色诊疗技术的调查、挖掘整理、研究评价及推广应用。

3. 强化中医药师承教育。建立中医药师承教育培养体系,将师承教育全面融入院校教育、毕业后教育和继续教育。

(四)着力推进中医药创新

1. 健全中医药协同创新体系。健全以国家和省级中医药科研机构为核心,以高等院校、医疗机构和企业为主体,以中医科学研究基地(平台)为支撑,完善中医药领域科技布局。

2. 加强中医药科学研究。探索适合中药特点的新药开发新模式,推动重大新药创制。

3.建立和完善符合中医药特点的科研评价标准和体系,研究完善有利于中医药创新的激励政策。

(五)全面提升中药产业发展水平

1.加强中药资源保护利用。

2.推进中药材规范化种植养殖。建立完善中药材原产地标记制度。

3.实施中药绿色制造工程,形成门类丰富的新兴绿色产业体系。

4.构建现代中药材流通体系,加强第三方检测平台建设。

(六)大力弘扬中医药文化

1.繁荣发展中医药文化。大力倡导"大医精诚"理念,推动中医药文化国际传播。

2.推动中医药与文化产业融合发展,探索将中医药文化纳入文化产业发展规划。

(七)积极推动中医药海外发展

1.加强中医药对外交流合作。实施中医药海外发展工程,推动中医药技术、药物、标准和服务走出去,促进国际社会广泛接受中医药。

2.扩大中医药国际贸易,加强中医药知识产权国际保护,扩大中医药服务贸易国际市场准入。

四、"健康中国2030"规划纲要(Outline of the "Healthy China 2030" Plan)

2016年10月25日,中共中央、国务院印发了《"健康中国2030"规划纲要》并发出通知,要求各地区各部门结合实际认真贯彻落实。

《"健康中国2030"规划纲要》第九章提出要充分发挥中医药独特优势。

(一)提高中医药服务能力

实施中医临床优势培育工程,强化中医药防治优势病种研究,加强中西医结合,提高重大疑难病、危急重症临床疗效。

(二)发展中医养生保健治未病服务

实施中医治未病健康工程,将中医药优势与健康管理结合,探索融健康文化、健康管理、健康保险为一体的中医健康保障模式。

(三)推进中医药继承创新

发展中医药健康服务,加快打造全产业链服务的跨国公司和国际知名的中国品牌,推动中医药走向世界。建立大宗、道地和濒危药材种苗繁育基地,提供中药材市场动态监测信息,促进中药材种植业绿色发展。

五、"十四五"中医药信息化发展规划(The "14th Five-Year Plan" for the Development of Traditional Chinese Medicine Informatization)

"十四五"时期,信息化进入加快数字化发展、建设数字中国的新阶段。习近平总书记强调,没有信息化就没有现代化。信息化为中华民族带来了千载难逢的机遇,是引领中医药传承创新发展的先导力量,为贯彻新发展理念,抢抓信息革命机遇,加快信息化建设,激发中医药行业新发展活力,为实施健康中国战略、推动中医药振兴发展提供强力支撑。2022 年 11 月 25 日,根据《中华人民共和国国民经济和社会发展第十四个五年规划和 2035 年远景目标纲要》《"十四五"国家信息化规划》《"十四五"中医药发展规划》《"十四五"推进国家政务信息化规划》《"十四五"全民健康信息化规划》等文件精神,国家中医药管理局制定了《"十四五"中医药信息化发展规划》,其主要任务概括如下。

(一)夯实中医药信息化发展基础

1. 加快信息基础设施提档升级。鼓励各级中医医疗机构规范接入区域全民健康信息平台,探索构建与区域全民健康信息平台互联互通的中医药信息平台。

2. 强化网络和数据安全防护。推进落实关键信息基础设施保护、等级保护、数据分类分级安全管理、个人隐私保护、安全审查和应急处置等各项工作,全面提升中医药行业安全保障能力。

3. 推进中医药信息标准应用。积极参与国际标准化组织和世界卫生组织的标准化活动,提升参与中医药信息国际标准化活动的能力。

(二)深化数字便民惠民服务

1. 加强中医医院智慧化建设。鼓励各地开展智慧中医医院建设,鼓励各地研发应用中医电子病历、名老中医传承信息系统、中医智能辅助诊疗系统等中医药特色系统,推广智慧中药房等服务模式。

2. 推动中医药健康服务与互联网深度融合。建设中医互联网医院,发展远程医疗和互联网诊疗,推动构建覆盖诊前、诊中、诊后的线上线下一体化中医医疗服务模式。

3. 优化中医馆健康信息平台。继续推进中医馆健康信息平台建设,强化业务功能一体化集成,持续完善中医药知识库和视频课程内容,增强中医适宜技术、中药处方的智能推荐。

4. 鼓励中医医院牵头组建的城市医疗集团、县域医共体开展智慧化建设,统一建设部署医院管理、医疗服务等信息平台,发挥移动互联网、大数据等在分级诊疗中的作用,推动中医医疗信息共享和服务协同。

(三)加强中医药数据资源治理

1. 强化中医药政务服务和管理。推动行政管理业务网上办理,推进业务流程优化、行政管理模式创新,促进线上线下业务融合发展。

2.贯彻实施国家中医药综合统计制度,加快建设制度完善、方法科学、过程可控的中医药综合统计体系。

3.建设中医药综合统计信息平台。

4.推动中医药统计数据开放共享,开展深度分析挖掘,建立统计数据定期发布机制,稳步推动数据资源共享开放。

（四）推进中医药数据资源创新应用

1.加快中医药关键数字技术攻关。利用大数据、人工智能等新一代信息技术加强名老中医学术经验、老药工传统技艺等活态传承,支持中医学术流派发展。

2.助力中药质量控制水平提升。推进中药材、中药饮片、中成药信息化追溯体系建设,基本实现中药重点品种来源可查、去向可追、责任可究。

3.创新中医药数字教育新模式。推动中医药在线开放教育资源和移动教育应用软件开发,开设在线课堂和远程学堂。

4.推动中医药文化数字化建设。鼓励中医药机构将中医药文化资源数据采集、加工、挖掘与数据服务纳入经常性工作。

六、"十四五"中医药人才发展规划(The "14th Five-Year Plan" for the Development of Traditional Chinese Medicine Talents)

为深入贯彻习近平总书记关于中医药工作的重要论述,落实中央人才工作会议、全国中医药大会以及第四届国医大师和第二届全国名中医表彰大会精神,加快中医药人才队伍建设,以高质量人才队伍推动中医药振兴发展,根据《中共中央国务院关于促进中医药传承创新发展的意见》《"十四五"中医药发展规划》《关于加强新时代中医药人才工作的意见》等文件要求,2022年10月14日,国家中医药管理局特制定本规划。

《"十四五"中医药人才发展规划》的主要任务有:第一,加强中医药高层次人才队伍建设。壮大中医药领军人才。在中医药高层次人才培养计划中设立青年专项。建立健全对青年人才的普惠性支持措施,改善青年人才成长环境,推动中医药青年人才快速成长。集聚多学科交叉创新人才,培养高层次中西医结合人才。第二,加强基层中医药人才队伍建设,提高毕业生下沉基层服务意愿,提升基层人才服务能力。加强中医馆骨干人才培训,加强中医医师队伍建设。推动各级中医医疗机构加强中医医师培养培训,通过进修、访学等形式,提升中医医师服务能力。加强中药师队伍建设。加强国家中医药优势特色教育培训基地能力建设,持续开展中药特色技术传承骨干人才培训项目。建设一批中医护理重点学科,培养中医护理学科带头人和骨干人才。加强中医技师队伍及少数民族医药人才队伍建设。第三,统筹加强其他重点领域中医药人才培养。培养中医药急需紧缺人才。鼓励建立各级中医药健康服务人员培训基地,面向健康服务行业人员开展中医药技术技能培训。培养中医药管理人才。持续实施中医医院院长职业化培训项目,实现地级市以上的中医类医院院长培训基本全覆盖。培养中医药文化和国际化人才。持续实施中医药文化传播行动,培养一批中医药文化科普传播专业人才。培养中医药师资人才。培养中医药标准化人才。深化中医药教育改革。健全中医药毕业后教育。推进中医药继续教育,扩大中医药继续教育项目可及性。深化中医药师承教育,培养一批中医临床人才。

七、关于加快中医药特色发展的若干政策措施(Policy Measures for Accelerating the Development of Traditional Chinese Medicine)

进一步落实《中共中央国务院关于促进中医药传承创新发展的意见》和全国中医药大会部署,遵循中医药发展规律,认真总结中医药防治新型冠状病毒感染经验做法,破解存在的问题,更好发挥中医药特色和比较优势,推动中医药和西医药相互补充、协调发展。2021年1月22日,国务院办公厅提出如下7条政策措施。

(一)夯实中医药人才基础

1.提高中医药教育整体水平。

2.坚持发展中医药师承教育。长期坚持推进名老中医药专家学术经验继承、优秀中医临床人才研修、传承工作室建设等项目。

3.加强中医药人才评价和激励。将中医药学才能、医德医风作为中医药人才主要评价标准,将会看病、看好病作为中医医师的主要评价内容。

(二)提高中药产业发展活力

1.优化中药审评审批管理。建立科技、医疗、中医药等部门推荐符合条件的中药新药进入快速审评审批通道的有效机制。

2.完善中药分类注册管理。尊重中药研发规律,完善中药注册分类和申报要求。充分利用数据科学等现代技术手段,建立中医药理论、人用经验、临床试验"三结合"的中药注册审评证据体系,积极探索建立中药真实世界研究证据体系。优化古代经典名方中药复方制剂注册审批。

(三)增强中医药发展动力

1.保障落实政府投入。落实对公立中医医院基本建设、设备购置、重点学科发展、人才培养等政府投入政策。

2.多方增加社会投入,打造中医药健康服务高地和学科、产业集聚区。

3.加强融资渠道支持,鼓励金融机构创新金融产品,支持中医药特色发展。

(四)完善中西医结合制度

1.创新中西医结合医疗模式。

2.健全中西医协同疫病防治机制。中医药系统人员第一时间全面参与公共卫生应急处置,中医药防治举措全面融入应急预案和技术方案。

3.完善西医学习中医制度。高职临床医学专业中开设中医基础与适宜技术必修课程。

4.提高中西医结合临床研究水平。

（五）实施中医药发展重大工程

1.实施中医药特色人才培养工程。加强高校附属医院、中医规范化培训基地等人才培养平台建设。

2.加强中医医疗服务体系建设。加强中医医院感染科、肺病科、发热门诊、可转换传染病区、可转换重症监护室等建设。

3.加强中医药科研平台建设。围绕中医理论、中药资源、中药创新、中医药疗效评价等重点领域建设国家重点实验室。

4.实施名医堂工程。国医大师、名老中医、岐黄学者等名医团队入驻名医堂的,实行创业扶持、品牌保护、自主执业、自主运营、自主培养、自负盈亏综合政策,打造一批名医团队运营的精品中医机构。

5.实施中医药产学研医政联合攻关工程。

6.制定中药材采收、产地初加工、生态种植、野生抚育、仿野生栽培技术规范,推进中药材规范化种植,鼓励发展中药材种植专业合作社和联合社。

7.建设国家中医药综合改革示范区,加快建立健全中医药法规、发展政策举措、管理体系、评价体系和标准体系。

8.制定"十四五"中医药"一带一路"发展规划,发展"互联网+中医药贸易",为来华接受中医药服务人员提供签证便利。

（六）提高中医药发展效益

1.完善中医药服务价格政策,完善分级定价政策。

2.健全中医药医保管理措施。探索符合中医药特点的医保支付方式,发布中医优势病种,鼓励实行中西医同病同效同价。

3.合理开展中医非基本服务。

（七）营造中医药发展良好环境

1.加强中医药知识产权保护。制定中药领域发明专利审查指导意见,进一步提高中医药领域专利审查质量,推进中药技术国际专利申请。

2.优化中医药科技管理,加强中医药科技活动规律研究,推进中医药科技评价体系建设。

3.切实加强中医药文化宣传,使中医药成为群众促进健康的文化自觉。在中华优秀传统文化传承发展工程中增设中医药专项。实施中医药文化传播行动,持续开展中小学中医药文化教育,打造中医药文化传播平台及优质产品。

4.提高中医药法治化水平。

第三节　中医药文化认同的研究现状
(Research Status of Cultural Identity of Traditional Chinese Medicine)

目前,国外关于中医药文化认同的研究尚为空白,相关成果限于国内且数量较少,主要涉及中医药文化认同的定义、作用、院校横断面调查及提升策略研究4个方面。

一、中医药文化认同定义研究(Research on the Definition of Cultural Identity of Traditional Chinese Medicine)

潘小毅等将中医药文化认同定义为有意识或无意识状态下向个人灌输的具有中医药文化属性的知识、信念、情感、行为、价值观等方面的个体感知。薛芳芸等认为中医药文化认同是指从心理认知、内在情感、思想观念和外在行为诸多方面肯定并赞同中医药文化,最终反映在行为上。李春提出中医药文化认同是对中医文化中精神层面包括医学观念、诊疗心理、道德伦理等要素的共识与认可,是将对人类思维行为起支配作用的中医药价值取向。吴晶晶等指出中医药文化认同是个体对群体组织灌输传递的含有中医药文化倾向的价值感知。

二、中医药文化认同作用研究(Research on the Influence of Cultural Identity of Traditional Chinese Medicine)

王雷等认为高度的中医药文化认同感将有利于学生更好地掌握中医知识、应用中医技能,将中医药文化真正作用于日常生活健康保障之中。吴晶晶等提出中医药文化认同的形成有助于个体学习与发展传统中医药文化,有助于中医药文化建设力度的加大与提升。另有汪永锋等认为中医药文化认同的培养是大力推进中医药国际化教育的基础。

三、中医药文化认同现状调查研究(Research on the Current Situation of Cultural Identity of Traditional Chinese Medicine)

韩凯莉等以问卷和访谈形式对全国多所非中医药院校大学生的中医药文化认同情况进行调查,对大学生关于中医药文化在认知程度、情感维度、行为付诸做差异化分析;结果表明,83.6%的非中医药院校大学生对于中医药文化认知度较低,但对于中医药文化的情感认同与行为付诸都有较高的积极性。罗中华等在一项研究中以甘肃省各级医疗机构在职医生为总体,通过随机抽样问卷调查发现,甘肃省医生对中医的认同水平较高,且认同水平存在差异,具体表现在年龄、职称、学历、医疗机构类型及地区分布方面。郑晓红等研究发现,大众对中医药文化核心价值的认同度总体较低,且与年龄、性别、受教育程度、职业及地区相关。然而王雷的研究发现,中医药文化核心价值的认同程度和年龄并不显著相关,但在学历、职业方面呈现出显著差异。

四、中医药文化认同提升策略研究(Research on Strategies for Promoting Cultural Identity of Traditional Chinese Medicine)

多数学者在各自研究中都进行了关于如何构建和提升中医药文化认同的讨论,且多从跨文化认同角度展开。王玮娇等系统归纳总结来华中医药留学生教育取得的成就与不足,并提出重视来华中医药留学生的战略作用,精心组织教学,提升其中医药文化认知水平,营造校园中医药文化氛围,扩大中医药文化宣传,强化留学生的临床实践,加深留学生对中医药的理解,提高来华中医药留学生教育供给能力等提升来华中医药留学生对中医药文化认同的策略。李春燕建议在文化全球化背景下通过"发掘、重构、输出"的三步走策略提高世界对中医药文化的认同,并指出提高中医药文化认同度的前提是要加强中医药文化自觉,完成在继承中实现中医药文化创新,争取在和"他者"文化的协调中提升中医药文化的张力。周铮亦从三方面总结了促进中医药跨文化认同的策略思路,强调首先要明确和保持中医药文化本真性,以此为基础在多元文化交融的过程中输送自身合理、优异的特质,如独特的认知方式、思维角度及融洽的伦理关系等。在这些对策中,"文化自觉""文化本真性"以及"文化输出"均被提及,对此后续研究也大多是在观照到这一点的基础上继续展开解决中医药文化认同问题的策略讨论。张宗明在总结中医药文化基因内容之后,强调要通过传承中医药文化基因来培养中医学子文化自信、提高中医工作者文化自觉、提升民众中医药文化认同感,以化解中医药文化认同危机。乔宁宁讨论了中医药文化身份的建构及其在跨文化传播中的价值适应问题,认为可以尝试将西医对中医的文化认同转变为中医在西医文化语境中的价值适应,从异域文化寻找自我的认同并予以强化,以此为传播策略促进中医药文化在全球范围取得更多理解与认同。

第二章
中医药文化历史与现状
(History and Current Researches of Traditional Chinese Medicine Culture)

文化兴国运兴,文化强民族强。没有高度的文化自信,就没有文化的繁荣兴盛,更不能实现中华民族的伟大复兴。中医药文化是中华民族优秀传统文化中体现中医药本质与特色的精神文明和物质文明的总和,培养中医文化自信是推动中医药事业的发展、扩大中华文化影响力的必然要求。通过学习中医药起源、发展及其当代价值,可以帮助人们了解中医药文化历史,学习中医文化内涵,引起人们对中医药文化的重视,培养中医药文化自信。

Culture promotes national prosperity. The powerful culture, the strong nation. Without the strong cultural confidence, there can be no thriving and prosperous culture, let alone the great rejuvenation of the Chinese nation. Traditional Chinese medicine culture is the sum of spiritual civilization and material civilization that embody the essence and characteristics of traditional Chinese medicine in the excellent culture of the Chinese nation. Cultivating confidence in traditional Chinese medicine culture is an inevitable requirement to promote Chinese medicine development and expand the its influence. By studying the origin, development, and contemporary value of traditional Chinese medicine, we aim to help people understand the cultural history of traditional Chinese medicine, learn the cultural connotations of traditional Chinese medicine, arouse people's attention to traditional Chinese medicine culture, and cultivate their confidence in traditional Chinese medicine culture.

第一节　中医药文化溯源
(Tracing the Origin of Traditional Chinese Medicine Culture)

一、中医药文化内涵(Cultural Connotation of Traditional Chinese Medicine)

文化是一个国家与民族的灵魂,是铸牢中华民族共同体意识的根本精神依托和深厚的思想资源。中医药文化是中华优秀传统文化中不可或缺的重要组成部分,是中国文化软实力的重要标签,作为中华优秀传统文化的重要组成部分,中医药文化集中体现了中华民族的核心价值、思维方式。

中医药学是中华民族几千年来在生产生活与疾病斗争中所逐步总结形成的医学科学体系,通过望、闻、问、切进行系统的诊断,全面地阐述了人体生理、病理以及疾病的诊断、治疗和养生保健,形成了其独特的理论框架,讲究"阴阳五行、天人合一、整体观念、辨证论治",蕴含着中华民族深邃的哲学思想。

中医药文化是中华民族优秀传统文化中体现中医药本质与特色的精神文明和物质文明的总和。中医药文化有广义和狭义之分,广义中医药文化是中医药物质文明和精神文明的总和,包括中医药的精神心理文化、行为制度文化、物质形象文化3个层面;狭义中医药文化特指中医药学的精神心理文化。中医药文化的基础是中国传统哲学、文学、史学,它由中医药精神文化、行为文化、物质文化3个方面构成,包含中医药文化理念、文化实践、文化环境3个层面,体现了中医药的人文属性。

二、从神话传说看中医药文化(Traditional Chinese Medicine Culture in Mythology and Legends)

原始社会人们因生产力低下、认知局限,对自然界的风雨雷电、日月更替等各种自然现象都无法解释,只能通过幻想的方式对自然界和社会形态进行艺术加工,把自然力加以形象化,借助想象以征服自然力,支配自然力,于是产生了崇拜自然的意识,人们渴望能够认识自然、征服自然、成为自然的主人,由于认知能力有限,人们只能将自然界各种变化归结于神的意志和统治,幻想自然现象背后有神灵的支配,于是从而产生万物有灵的观念,如此由自然崇拜过渡到神灵崇拜。

神话是先民们用想象和幻想的形式对当时无法解释的各种现象进行的拟人化的解释,神话和传说虽然是对想象的不切实际的表达,但体现了人类征服和改造自然的积极意义,反映了我国古代人类思维发展的原始状况。人们可以从神话中找到哲学的、宗教的、伦理的、美学的,甚至科学的萌芽,也可从中看到历史的折射、社会的结构、思维的演化。神话从某种程度上也可以反映出当时的历史文化,广为流传的神话故事有女娲补天、夸父追日、精卫填海等,其中神农尝百草是最具有医学特色的神话。

神农不仅是农耕社会的鼻祖,也是中医中药最早开拓者。远古时期,百姓以采食野生瓜果、生吃动物蚌蛤为生,经常有人受毒害得病死亡,因此人民寿命普遍较短。炎帝神农氏为"宣药疗疾"使百姓益寿延年,他跋山涉水,行遍三湘大地,尝遍百草,了解百草之平毒寒温之药性。为了找寻治病解毒良药,他几乎嚼尝过所有植物,"日遇七十毒"。神农在尝百草的过程中,识别了百草,发现了具有攻毒祛病、养生保健作用的中药。由此令民有所"就",不复为"疾病",故先民封他为"药神",炎帝神农氏终因误尝断肠草而死,葬于长沙茶乡之尾。

被誉为我国神话之渊府的《山海经》一书保存了有关我国上古时代民族、宗教、历史、地理、医药、生物、矿产等宝贵而丰富的资料,是我国古代的百科全书,是研究我国上古社会的重要文献。其中《山海经》中详细记载的医学资料、医药知识为研究远古时代医学的发展和演变提供了宝贵资料。

《山海经》记载了包括内科、外科、五官科及预防医学的 50 余种疾病的症状,有些还被后世中医所采纳,如疠、痈、疽、瘕、痔、癣、瘘、蛊、疟、瘿等已成为中医学的专用术语。据统计,《山海经》全书共记 124 种药物,这些药物可细分为植物药、动物药和矿物药(包括化石类药物),药物的使用方式多样,主要有服、食、佩、席、乘等,反映了中医药用药途径的原始风貌。有些药物与其对应治疗的疾病一起出现,有些药物则并非用于疗疾,而是具有养生、美容或医学方面的其他神奇功效,有些药物具有综合功效,可以治疗两种及以上疾病或兼具疗疾和其他功效。《山海经》中所记载的药物虽然表象、来源甚至疗效都经过虚妄的想象与联想,但其原型并非凭空捏造,而是真实存在,甚至确具相应功效,这一点在历代本草典籍的记录与中医学的临证实践中可获得验证。《山海经》所载的药物功效,一般均一药治一病,少数兼治两种疾病。这表明祖国的中药文化从单味应用到复方配伍,以至后来系统的配伍理论都是经历了漫长的进化历程。

三、宗教巫术与医的萌芽(Religious Witchcraft and the Emergence of Medicine)

众所周知,远古时代社会生产力极其低下,人们对千变万化的自然现象无法解释,于是将无法解释的自然现象赋予一个名称"灵魂",认为万物皆有灵魂,将世界划分成能看到摸到的现实世界、看不见摸不到的神灵世界两部分,将人的伤病死亡或康复都归结于鬼神控制。为了保证部落群体的生存和发展,就要处理好人和鬼神的关系,人们因此通过祭祀、歌舞、占卜等方式对鬼神进行祈福,祈求平安,从而形成了初步的巫术。最早的巫术是自发形成的,不以牟利骗人为动机。在当时巫术包括了全部的文化要素,当然也包括医术在内,巫师一般较为聪明,拥有歌唱、舞蹈、表演、绘画、祭祀等多种知识和技能。巫师具备相应的学识,了解治病的草药,有时会让患者服用一些草药或矿物,寓意让神灵去制服致病的鬼神,驱走恶魔,祈求健康,也成了最早意义上的医生。

在巫术疗法处于统治地位的时代,人们的医药知识也在日益增长,人们在日常生活中凭借自己的经验发现一些动植物、矿物的属性,此类的经验日益积累形成了最早的医药知识。据史书记载,中国最早的医人皆为巫。《说文解字》称"古者巫彭初作医",相传巫彭就是医术的发明者,巫彭是以巫之身份侧重于行医的名巫,此期巫术中的医术具有一定的独立性,但医药领域尚未形成理论体系,没有揭示药物与疾病的本质联系,此时仍呈现出半医半巫的状态。

随着生产力的不断发展进步、社会的剧烈变动,医和巫在春秋时期开始出现明显的斗争,在思想上科学与迷信、唯物主义和唯心主义的斗争也日益尖锐。医学的发展水平也已初步具备了向巫术挑战与之决裂的资本,医学的唯物主义倾向日益明显,春秋末代和战国年代,医家将五行、阴阳等理论引入医学体系。扁鹊提出病有六不治,其中有一条是凡信巫不信医的不治,这可能是中国医学史上巫和医开始分家的第一个独立宣言。《黄帝内经》在总结医药知识和临床经验的基础上,以阴阳、五行思想为指导,构建了较为完善科学的中医学理论体系基础,书中明确指出了医术和巫术相互对立、不可调和,标志着医巫两者的解体。从此医学逐渐冲破它的羁绊,确立了自己的独立地位,走上科学发展的道路。

四、中医用具起源(Origin of Traditional Chinese Medicine Appliances)

针灸是祖国传统医药学伟大宝库的重要组成部分,当前全球已有 183 个国家和地区应用针灸,针灸已然成为中医药走向世界的名片,其影响力对促进中医药和中国文化的国际传播具有重要意义。针灸起源于原始社会的新石器时代,距今已有 5000 ~ 8000 年,而实际上其发端可追溯到数万年乃至数十万年前的旧石器时代。远古时期的人们由于经常受伤,创口常发生溃疡化脓,疼痛难以忍受时人们发现用一些尖锐的石器刺破伤口,伤口流脓会减轻疼痛同时加速愈合,头、四肢疼痛时,用石头去敲打某个部位反而会产生减轻疼痛的效果,于是当时人们发生某些病痛或不适的时候,不自觉地用手按摩、捶拍,用尖锐的石器按压疼痛不适的部位,而使原有的症状减轻或消失,应时而生出最早的针具——砭石。

砭石可谓是最古老的医疗器械和外科手术工具的起源,除了用于化脓性感染地切开排脓外,还用于刺病和放血。古代对砭针的石材很有讲究,并非任何粗糙的石头均可磨成砭针,必须选择结构严密和纹理细腻的石材才可以磨成砭针。《山海经·东山经》有这样的记载:"高氏之山,其上多玉,其下多箴(针)石。"在金属针产生以前,人们也曾运用过骨针、陶针、竹针、木针等,但这些都是过渡性的,使用并不普遍。随着生产力的发展,冶金技术的发明,金属逐渐被人们用来制造生产工具,这为制造金属针提供了前提条件,促进了针刺用具的进一步改进,青铜针、金针、银针、铁针相继问世。砭石逐渐被金属针具取代,从而扩大了针刺的应用范围,加快了针灸术的发展进程。

灸法的起源离不开火的发现和使用,早在旧石器时代,人类就掌握了火的使用,将火运用于灸疗也同样起源于新石器时代。起初人类在使用火取暖的过程中发现用火进行局部的灼烤不仅可以御寒,还可以缓解由于着凉受寒引起的关节疼痛,用兽皮包裹着灼热的石块贴敷在身体既舒适又保暖,最早的热熨技术也由此形成。在不断地经验积累过程中人们发现用艾蒿一类药科植物燃烧进行灼烤的效果最好,于是将艾灸疗法定型下来,不断加以改进和规范化,因而形成了比较成熟的艾灸疗法。

拔罐法的出现比灸法晚,拔罐是借助热力排除罐中空气,利用负压使其吸着于皮肤,造成瘀血现象的一种治病方法。这种疗法可以逐寒祛湿、疏通经络、祛除淤滞、行气活血、消肿止痛、拔毒泻热,具有调整人体的阴阳平衡、解除疲劳、增强体质的功能,从而达到扶正祛邪、治愈疾病的目的。我国有关拔罐最早的记载见于春秋战国时期的医籍《五十二病方》,书中提到了用"角"来治病,书中提到用角细小的前端来对准病患部位,吸取痔疮需要割除的地方,此时的角是人们通过狩猎获取的野兽的角。后来随着科学的进步,经验的积累,在隋唐时期拔罐的工具得到了突破性的进展,人们开始用竹罐代替兽角,竹罐取材方便,价格低廉,容易获取,因此在民间得到广泛的推广和应用。在清代,拔罐疗法又获得了巨大的发展和创新,在理论上人们将拔罐疗法与脏腑经络学说相结合,扩大了拔罐的治疗范围,在拔罐器具上,人们发现竹罐的吸力较差且易爆裂漏气,人们尝试使用陶罐发现效果甚好,陶罐得到了广泛流传。随着工艺技术的不断发展进步,人们开始逐渐使用玻璃制罐,玻璃罐的优点是质地清晰透明,使用时观察所拔部位皮肤充血程度,便于随时掌握情况,且罐口光滑,吸拔力好,目前已被人们广泛应用。

五、中药发展(Development of Traditional Chinese Medicine)

中药学是中国传统药物学,1840 年以前统称为本草学,包括动物、植物、矿物药,种类数不胜数。关于中药的起源本源并没有详细的记载。《史记纲鉴》中记载"神农尝百草,始有医药",相传神农尝百草,一日遇七十毒,生动地反映出人们认识药物的艰难过程。在远古时代人类没有什么药物学的知识也不懂得区分有毒和无毒的物质,他们四处迁徙,走到哪里就吃当地的食物,很多时候会误食一些有毒甚至是剧毒的东西引起呕吐、腹泻、昏迷甚至死亡,也可能偶然进食一些食物使原来的病痛得到缓解从而发现有的植物尽管有毒但是适量食用也可以达到治疗疾病的效果。于是人们总结这些反复出现的情况逐步积累经验,形成了初步对药的认识。民间也一直流传着药食同源的说法,认为药是从食物中选择出来的,原始人受凉后出现恶寒、微热、头痛、喷嚏,服食了生姜、紫苏、葱之类食物后随着汗出而诸症缓解。以后经过反复试用就会用这类食物来治"风寒感冒"了。在咳嗽时吃了白果、杏仁、桃仁后症状缓解了,以后就渐渐会用之来治疗咳嗽。后来随着采矿业的发展,人们对矿物质的认识不断加深,使用中人们逐渐发现一些矿物质的性能,积累起了有关矿物药学的知识。

第二节　中医文化和中华文化
(Traditional Chinese Medicine Culture and Chinese Culture)

　　文化是一个民族的灵魂和血脉,是一个民族的标记和生存方式,是民族赖以生存和延续的根本。中华文化是中华各族人民在社会发展过程中所创造的物质文化和精神文化的总和,是中国人价值体系和生活方式的总和。百家争鸣的中国哲学、延绵不断的中国历史、底蕴丰富的中国语言、多姿多彩的传统手艺、效果显著的传统医学等构成了中国传统文化的基本内涵。在我国悠久的历史长河中,中医文化深深扎根于中华文化,汲取其哲学思想、人文历史、生命科学等优秀理论,形成了具有中华特色的中医文化理论体系。中医药文化是中华民族优秀传统文化中体现中医药本质与特色的精神文明和物质文明的总和。中医药事业是打开中医文化宝库的钥匙,中医药学凝聚着中华民族深邃的智慧体系,健康的养生理念和丰富的实践总结,是中华民族优秀文化的重要组成部分。中医药文化以其科学的理论体系、卓越的治疗效果为中华民族的繁衍昌盛和人类健康做出了不可磨灭的贡献。

　　中医文化是中华民族优秀文化的重要组成部分和杰出代表,中医学是在中华传统文化的背景下成长发展起来的。中国传统文化是儒、道、释三种流派思想长期融合而来的。儒学中的天人合一、以人为本、以和为贵、中庸等思想;道家的祸福相倚、对立统一、沉静无为等思想;佛教中的众生平等、慈悲为怀等思想均对中医学的形成与发展影响深远。尤其是强调人与自然界协调统一的"天人合一"观,不仅是中国传统文化的精髓之一,也直接缔造了中医学的基本框架,为中医学的起步与发展找到了出发点与归宿。中医天人相应的整体观念、五行相贯的藏象学说、阴阳互根的治疗原则无不打上了中国古代哲学的烙印。

一、古典中医和儒家(Classical Chinese Medicine and Confucianism)

　　中医学的理论体系是在传统哲学指导下经过长期临床实践逐步形成和发展起来的,它在春秋战国到秦汉之际就初具规模。儒学文化渗入到中医学中,对中医学产生了极为深刻的影响,在中医的理、法、方、药等方面都体现了儒家的思想。中庸,是儒家思想的核心体系之一,主要阐发于孔子《论语》:"中庸之为德也,其至矣乎?"(《雍也》)。《礼记·中庸》做了专门论述。中庸,即持中、适中、和谐,指不偏不倚。中庸的哲理主要体现在对待事物时把握其适度,这个度是事物与量的最佳限度。中庸绝不是折中主义,不是无原则地调和,中庸是一种较难掌握的、辩证地处理事物的准则。因此,可以说中庸是儒学哲理的活的灵魂。

儒家中庸的和谐观影响着中医的协调观,儒家的"中和"理念对中医的生理病理学有着深远的影响。从人体的生理过程看,"阴在内,阳之守也;阳在外,阴之使也"。中医学以阴阳平衡为人体生命活动的理想状态标志着人体健康,一旦这种协调被破坏,人体就会进入病理状态。中医学的"阴平阳秘"继承了儒家"中庸"的学术思想,中医学在生理上强调"阴平阳秘"。疾病的发生,从根本上说是阴阳的相对平衡遭到破坏,即阴阳的偏盛或偏衰代替了正常的阴阳消长,《黄帝内经》就是用这种对立统一失其平衡造成阴阳偏盛偏衰的理论,来进一步解释寒、热、虚、实等病理变化的,主张诊治疾病要平调阴阳,使患者机体内环境达到阴阳动态平衡,从而达到疾病痊愈。"辨证论治"是中医学理论体系的特征之一,也是对儒家思想"允执其中"的进一步发挥和体现。

儒家"仁爱"思想为古典中医的医德医风奠定道德基础。"仁"是儒家道德思想体系中最完美、最高尚的人格境界,是古代知识阶层共同追求的人生目标,孔子确立了"仁"学思想体系,其基本含义是"爱人"。首先是爱自己的亲人即以"孝悌"为"仁之本",继而以忠恕之道将这种血缘关系推广至社会上所有的人即"泛爱众",要求爱一切的人。"仁"是儒家思想的核心,中医学者将这一道德理念融入医学领域中并在中医学领域发挥其独特内涵,认为医学不仅仅是医疗技术的运用更赋予医学以道德属性。《古今医统大全》中"医以活人为心,故曰医乃仁术",近似于当今医界所提倡的"仁心仁术",要求医生以仁爱之心,施以精湛的医术,拯救生命。

二、古典中医和道教(Classical Chinese Medicine and Taoism)

道教,产生于东汉中叶,至今已有1800年历史了,它以"道"为最高信仰,道教认为"道具有永恒的生命",获得保持它可以达到长生,这也成为"德"。道教追求安乐和长生,蕴含着积极的重人贵生的人生观念,正是这样的思想文化环境积淀了中国几千年重人生的思想观念,并且给以人为中心的道教和中医文化奠定思想基础,在漫长的历史发展中,道教和中医相互影响。

道教的养生家认为要做到长生不老就要爱护保养自己的躯体,只有通过自身的保养和修炼才可以获得生命的长存。养性,道家称之为性功,养性即为养心,心与性本为一体,不宜强分,养性亦为养心,炼心所以炼性。《庄子》提出的"心斋""坐忘",《太平经》中的"存神""守中"都与养性有很大的关系。道家认为养性的同时可以涵养道德,认为人的是非好恶都是由欲望引起的,主张人要节情寡欲。中医也十分注重养生,重人性命,中医情志养生始于《黄帝内经》,又于后世逐步发展,其间受道家思想影响颇多。道家提倡"少私寡欲""清静无为",这些思想构成了道家养神、宁神的摄生观,也渗透到中医情志养生中。

中医学从道家养性思想中汲取精华,与医学的特点相互结合发展,形成了调摄情志的观点,并将其理论运用到养生防治康复锻炼的领域,并且赋予其新的内容。中医对人类的情志做了更加细致、具体的分类和研究。《素问·阴阳应象大论篇》中言:"人有五脏化五气,以生喜怒悲忧恐。"《素问·上古天真论篇》也提出:"恬淡虚无,真气从之,精神内守,病安从来。"可见道家的精神调养基本奠定了中医情志养生的思想基调。中医认为人的七情各具特征,相互又有质的差别,因此其治病程度又有轻重、缓急、多少的不同。关于情志调摄的方法,中医注重清净修心养神,这与道家的说法颇为相近,如《黄帝内经》中提出了"恬淡虚无"的观点。

中医接受了道家哲学的本体生成论和一元观,并首先将自己的理论在关于人之生命的哲学方面做了定位。《素问·生气通天论》说:"自古通天者,生之本,本于阴阳。"认为人的生命是宇宙生成的一个环节,并与整个宇宙息息相关,它所依赖的根本就在于阴阳。在道家本体生存论和一元观的指导下,中医组建了自己完备的、有关人之生命的理论。由上可知,在中医学发展的历史实践中,道学对中医学理论的形成和发展起到了非常重要的作用,中医是道教养生的集大成者,秉承了道统思想,遵循人体系统的运行规律,人体和外部环境的交互影响,辨证施治,自然养生,道教学对中医学的贡献毋庸置疑。

三、古典中医与佛教(Classical Chinese Medicine and Buddhism)

佛教起源于古印度,创始人为释迦牟尼。2500多年以来,佛教广泛传播于世界很多国家和地区,两汉时期,佛教传入中国。佛教虽然发源于古印度,但至魏晋之后逐渐中国化,对中国的社会和文化生活产生广泛而深远的影响,成为我国传统文化不可忽视的重要组成部分。中医基础理论是中医学的核心部分,自佛教传入便与其结下不解之缘。两者在漫长的发展过程中相互渗透、相互补充,为中华民族的健康与繁衍做出了不可磨灭的历史贡献。

自东汉始,印度医药随佛教传入我国。魏晋时大量佛经被译成汉文,六朝时,中医学受印度医学影响较大,已有医书收载佛医药。唐代是中国佛教最兴盛的时期,佛医学理论、方药大量进入中国,并被一些中国医家所吸收,佛医文献是我国医学宝库中重要的组成部分。在孙思邈的《千金要方》和《千金翼方》中,就有十多个来自天竺的药方,诸如阿伽陀圆主万病方、婆罗门按摩法、服菖蒲方等等。佛教经典中的治疗药物大多为草类、木类、矿物类,其中龙脑、木香、豆蔻、乳香、没药、郁金、诃黎勒、返魂香等数十种药物,原产于印度、西域、东南亚等地,伴随佛教传入我国,成为中药的重要组成部分。

佛法思想具有明显的辩证思维特征,佛教反对各种片面、独断或绝对的理论和思维方法,佛教认为人有四万八千种病症,因此有四万八千种法门来应对,不同的病症应用不同的方法来救治。中医同样也注重辨证论治,如"异病同治""同病异治"等,其基本内涵就是治病求本,以人为本。佛教中的"四大"理论也对中医理论的基础产生了一定的影响,《佛医经》云:"人身中本有四病,一者地,二者水,三者火,四者风。风增气起,火增热起,水增寒起,土增力盛","四大不调,四百四病同时俱作","地水火风共成身,随彼因缘招异果"。在孙思邈《千金方》中也说:"凡四气合德,四神安和,一气不调,百一病生,四神同作,四百四病,同时俱发。"南北朝陶弘景增补《肘后方》序云:"人用四大成身,一大辄有一百一病。"从这些著作中都可以看出佛教思想的影响。佛教的"烦恼观念"对中医养生思想影响比较明显,佛教饮食倡导的"戒杀""素食"等饮食观念对中医食疗学产生了一定的影响。

中医药学也称"仁术",仁爱精神为中医医德的核心内容,佛教盛行之后,佛教的"戒律"对中医医德的发展也产生了一定的影响。戒律中最重要的是五戒,在五戒之中,不杀生又是位居榜首。"生"指一切有情生命,包括人类和所有动物。杀生的罪业是极重的,为十恶业之首,因此这种观念也或多或少影响到医家的思想。孙思邈在《大医精诚》这篇名著中说:"凡大医治病,必当安神定志,无欲无求,先发大慈恻隐之心,誓愿普救含灵之苦。"明代医家陈实功在其所著的《外科正宗》一书中也提出了类似戒律的"医家五戒十要"。总之,佛教思想中的"戒律"对正医风、立医德也起到了积极作用。

四、中医药文化与中国民俗(Traditional Chinese Medicine Culture and Chinese Folklore)

民俗是人类文化的重要组成部分,民俗的发展史也是人类文明化的历史,中医药学根植于中国传统民族文化的土壤,中国民俗文化中有许多习俗包含着中医药文化的思想,中医与民俗具有水乳交融的密切联系。

古代饮食习俗彰显中医药智慧。饮食文化最初可以追溯到旧石器时代,人类发现并学会使用火之后就告别了茹毛饮血的时代,走上了熟食的阶段。古代人从采集野果食用起就开始逐渐积累对食、药的认识,人们生病之后,偶然食用某种植物而痊愈,从而发现了某种食物的药性,在不断的实践和经验积累的过程中对药食同源的认识不断加深。例如彝族用鸡血治疗烧伤、用鹿骨治疗刀伤,鄂伦春族用鹿血拌红糖和黄酒治疗心悸等。民间关于饮食防病的习俗也有很多,立春是一年二十四节气中的第一个节气,立春揭开了春天的序幕。每年立春日,民间都有吃春饼的风俗,中医认为立春吃春饼对健康大有裨益。《素问·四气调神大论》指出:"春三月,此为发陈,天地俱生,万物以荣。"立春日是万物复苏的开始,这天起,阳气转盛,天气转暖,人体之阳气也要顺应自然,向上向外疏发,故中医讲究"春夏养阳"。春饼的原料主要是葱和韭菜,都是补阳食物,葱可以发汗解表、散寒通阳、杀菌解毒。我国无论是北方还是南方,在秋冬交替时,经常喜欢煮食鸭汤以抗寒气、防感冒，这是由于秋冬交替季节，寒气渐盛，而鸭肉具有助阳抗寒之功。清代《本经逢原》记载其"温中补虚，扶阳利水，是其本性。男子阳气不振者，食之最宜"，这些都是药食同源的具体表现。人们在长期的实践过程中积累了丰富的药食经验知识，经过历代医学名家整理完善又反过来指导人们的饮食习惯。

民俗活动具有养生保健意义。春天放风筝是中华民族的传统习俗，对人的身体健康非常有益。中医认为放风筝者沐浴在和煦的阳光和春风里，能"疏泄内热，舒筋活络"。《续博物志》也有"放风筝，张口仰视，可以泄热"之说。在明媚的春光里踏春放风筝，可以舒展筋骨，让身体随着放飞的风筝而不停移动，从而活动四肢，尽情呼吸新鲜空气，吐故纳新。中医也认为人类的生命活动具有运动的特征，因而积极提倡运动保健。《吕氏春秋·尽数》云："流水不腐，户枢不蠹，动也。形气亦然，形不动则精不流，精不流则气郁。"

第三节　中医药贡献
（Contributions of Traditional Chinese Medicine）

中国医学的历史是一部记录着中医药起源、形成与发展的巨著，是我国各族人民生产、生活以及同疾病斗争的经验总结。它从实践中来，又运用到实践中去。它的发展永无止境，从各个学科的不断进步中汲取营养，不断改革创新，不断开拓前行。中医药是中国医学体系的一个特色和优势，为中华民族的繁衍昌盛发挥了不可替代的作用，也为世界人民的健康事业做出了杰出贡献。随着医学模式的转变，已有越来越多的国家和地区关注中医药的发展。中医药学是中华优秀传统文化的重要组成部分，中医药从理论到丰富的实践，都是世界医学宝库的瑰宝。

在人类的历史长河中，中医一直是抗击疫情的重要力量。天花是由天花病毒引起的传染病，在天花存在的几千年里，它的传染性之强、肆虐范围之广、死亡率之高，可谓使人"闻之丧胆"，有史学家认为"人类史上最大的种族屠杀事件不全靠枪炮实现，而是天花"。而天花的消亡和人痘接种术的发明密不可分。人痘接种术始于我国明代，从痘衣法、痘浆法、旱痘法到改善的水苗法，种痘术也在不断地发展完善，较之英国人琴纳发明用牛痘苗预防天花早多年。另外有关阻断疫情，很早就提出过隔离检疫措施，以防止传染病的扩散。清嘉庆年间《海录》中就有记载，对外来海船实行海港检疫，以防止痘疮带入境内。

1954—1956年，我国部分地区乙型脑炎流行，应用温病学理论和方法的治疗取得了良好的效果。如石家庄地区采用白虎汤加味治疗，降低了乙型脑炎的病死率，提高了治愈率，减轻了后遗症，并得到医学界的认可，引起了广泛重视，在很大程度上纠正了中医不能治疗传染病的偏颇思想,也吸引了西医界不少有识之士投入中医学特别是温病学的学习和研究中。在 2003 年抗击"非典"疫情时,中医药疗法在减轻发热症状、控制病情进展、提高治愈率、缩短治疗时间、降低病亡率、减少并发症等方面成效明显,得到世界卫生组织的肯定。

屠呦呦:"青蒿素是中医药献给世界的礼物。"疟疾是世界上最主要的高死亡率传染病。20 世纪 60 年代,在氯喹抗疟失效、人类饱受疟疾之害的情况下,在中医研究院中药研究所任研究实习员的屠呦呦于 1969 年接受了国家疟疾防治项目"523"办公室艰巨的抗疟研究任务。屠呦呦担任中药抗疟组组长,研究小组从古代中药书籍和民间经验中梳理出近百种可能的抗疟疾中药,提取其中的有效成分。经过不断的研究与尝试,屠呦呦团队最终于 1972 年发现了青蒿素。青蒿素的发现,为世界带来了一种全新的抗疟药。以青蒿素为基础的联合疗法已经成为疟疾的标准治疗方法,在过去的 20 多年间,青蒿素联合疗法在全球疟疾流行地区广泛使用。据世卫组织不完全统计,青蒿素在全世界已挽救了数百万人的生命,每年治疗患者数亿人。

第三章

中医药智慧
(Wisdom of Traditional Chinese Medicine)

中医药是中国古代科学的瑰宝,凝聚着深邃的哲学智慧和中华民族几千年的健康养生理念及实践经验。中医药在历史发展进程中,兼容并蓄、创新开放,形成了独特的生命观、健康观、疾病观、防治观,实现了自然科学与人文科学的融合和统一,蕴含了中华民族深邃的哲学思想,形成了多种医家学派和医学理论,在人类健康文明史中熠熠生辉。随着人们健康观念变化和医学模式转变,应对全球卫生挑战、推进国际卫生合作、推动完善全球公共卫生治理,中医药越来越显示出其独特价值,必将日益发挥独特而重要的作用。

As a treasure of ancient Chinese science, traditional Chinese medicine embodies the profound philosophical wisdom and health preservation concepts for thousands of years and practical experiences of the Chinese nation. In the process of historical development, traditional Chinese medicine has been inclusive, innovative, creative and open to form a unique view on life, health, disease, prevention and treatment. It has achieved the integration and unity of natural science and humanities, has embodied the profound philosophical thinking of the Chinese nation, and has formed various medical schools and theories with shining brightly in the history of human health civilization. As people's health concepts and medical models change, traditional Chinese medicine (TCM) will be increasingly demonstrating its unique value to play a unique and important role in addressing global health challenges, promoting international health cooperation, and improving global public health governance.

第一节　中医四诊
(Four Diagnostic Methods in Traditional Chinese Medicine)

中医药作为中华文明的瑰宝,在抗击非典型性肺炎和新型冠状病毒感染疫情中都发挥了重要的作用,并做出了巨大的贡献。在中医药传承发展、守正创新的时代背景下,四诊作为中医诊断辨证的基础,在疾病诊疗中发挥着巨大作用,具备高效且准确的特点。

中医四诊包括望诊、闻诊、问诊和切诊四种,是在历代医家长期医疗实践的基础上逐步形成和发展起来,并随着时代的进步不断得到补充和完善的中医疾病诊察方法。①望诊是通过视觉观察患者的神、色、形、态、舌、排出物、小儿示指络脉等的异常变化,以了解病情的诊断方法。②闻诊是医生通过听觉和嗅觉,了解由患者病体发出的各种异常声音和气味,以诊察病情的方法,包括听声音和嗅气味两方面的内容。③问诊是医生通过询问患者或陪诊者,了解疾病的发生、发展、治疗经过、现在症状和其他与疾病有关的情况,以诊察疾病的方法。④切诊是医生用手指或手掌对患者的脉和全身特定或相关部位进行触、摸、按、叩,并通过手的触觉及患者的反应状态,以了解病情、诊察疾病的方法。

一、四诊基本内容(Basic Contents of Four Diagnostic Methods)

(一)基本程序与方法

望、闻、问、切四诊,分别从不同角度收集病情资料,在实际应用中应四诊并重,诸法参用。其具体操作多以问诊为先导,在问诊的过程中根据患者的具体情况,或先后,或交叉,分别进行望诊、闻诊及切诊,全面获取病情资料。对于医生诊察时不能直接获取的望诊、闻诊信息,可通过询问患者、陪诊者获取,或事后有条件时再获取、观察。

(二)基本要求

一般情况下,四诊操作应在安静、整洁、空气流通的诊室中进行,室内的温度、湿度、气压等要保持在舒适的范围内,尽量使医生各种感觉的敏感度少受影响;诊室应备有四诊操作所需要的物品和设备,如脉枕、手电筒、压舌板等;操作需患者暴露身体时,要注意保护其隐私;四诊操作最好选择在白天进行,晚间就诊的患者必要时可在白天再进行复诊。

(三)注意事项

1. 心身状态　让患者在心情平静、呼吸均匀、全身放松、主动配合的状态下接受检查;遇到患者不能配合进行某些操作,如神志昏迷、神乱、语言障碍、听力障碍、患者不愿意配合等情况,操作者可根据实际情况灵活掌握,尽可能地获取患者的信息。

2. 体位姿势　患者一般采取坐位或仰卧位,医生应根据诊察需要,指导患者改变体位或做出相应动作以配合检查。根据望诊、切诊需要,让患者充分暴露受检部位,并注意双侧对比等;切诊时,应让患者解除压迫被诊手臂的物件,如手表、挎包、扣紧的袖口等。

3. 着装打扮　医生应注意患者是否化妆、染发,或佩戴假肢及其他矫正肢体辅助器械,区分由于人为因素所致的改变。

4. 体内外环境　医生应注意年龄、性别、体质、种族、季节、昼夜、地理环境以及饮酒、饮食、药物、情绪、运动、日晒等体内外因素对面色、舌象、脉象等的影响。

(四)四诊的具体操作

1. 望诊　在开始接触患者的短暂时间内,首先对患者的整体状况(神气、面部色泽、形体及动态等）进行观察；在此基础之上，再根据病情诊断的需要，对患者的某些局部（如头面、颈项、躯体、四肢、二阴、皮肤等）情况及某些排出物（如痰、涎、涕、呕吐物、大小便等）的形、色、质、量等进行观察；常规情况下，对每位患者的舌象都要观察；对 3 岁以下的婴幼儿，还应注意观察患儿示指络脉的情况；望色泽时应注意排除各种体内、外因素所致色泽的生理性改变（如饮食、气温、情绪等）及人为因素所致改变（如染发、化妆等）；注意将患者色泽的变化与正常色泽进行比较。

2. 闻诊　医生与患者进行语言交流或体格检查时，应当仔细听患者所发之声音和嗅患者发出的气味。如遇患者有异常声音或气味的症状但当时无表现者，可通过询问患者及陪诊者而获取相关资料。

3. 问诊　临床上应根据就诊对象的具体情况，如初诊或复诊、急性疾病或慢性疾病等，对诊察过程中发现的问题及与疾病相关的问题进行系统、全面而有重点的询问。对于初诊的慢性病患者，首先询问主诉，其次围绕主诉对其现病史及既往史进行详细询问，必要时再对其家族史、个人史等进行询问；对于急性或危重疾病的患者，首先通过对患者或陪诊者的扼要询问，抓住主症，并进行重点检查，以迅速救治患者或缓解患者的病痛。待病情缓解或稳定后再对其他与病情相关的内容进行详细询问；对于反复就诊、已建立病案的患者，首先浏览其以往的就诊记录，了解其既往史及最近的病情，再询问本次就诊的问题或最近的病情变化及治疗效果等。

4. 切诊

（1）调息：医生调匀呼吸，宁静心神，全神贯注，可以通过自己的呼吸计算患者脉搏跳动的次数。

（2）指法

1）布指：医生用左手或右手的示指、中指与无名指诊脉。首先示指、中指与无名指的指端平齐，自然弯曲呈弓形，然后以中指确定关脉部位（高骨定关），示指按于关前的寸脉，无名指按于关后的尺脉，指目紧贴于脉动部位，与被诊者体表约呈 45°角。依据患者身高、臂长的差别调整布指的疏密。患者身高臂长者，布指宜疏，反之宜密。

2）一指定三关：对于儿童，运用左手或右手的拇指或示指总候三部，以掌后高骨定位，诊脉时用一指分别向两侧滑动或挪动的方式体察三部脉象。

3）运指：分别运用不同指力，采用轻取、中取、重取的方式，并依照先轻后重的顺序和视具体情况运用总按、单按、一指定三关等指法体察脉象。

（3）诊脉时间：每手诊脉时间不少于 1 分钟，两手以 3 分钟为宜，以体察可能发生的脉象变化。

二、四诊发展现状（Current Researches of Four Diagnostic Methods）

中医四诊作为中医诊断的基础方法，在临床中主要应用于各种疾病的诊断以及体质的辨识。但中医四诊要求医生在获取信息的基础上利用经验进行分析并做出准确判断,主观性强,对医生的要求较高,因此,中医四诊客观化成为发展方向。近年来,伴随着人工智能技术的快速发展,有学者借助自然语言处理、计算机视觉、知识图谱和深度学习等技术来促进中医四诊逐渐向着数据化、标准化、客观化乃至智能化的方向发展,针对中医四诊中的单项或四诊融合,从历史发展或临床诊断技术方面对其标准化和客观化进行了相关总结。

目前,中医四诊智能化研究的热点主要集中于舌诊、面诊、切诊、问诊方面。而闻诊中声诊和嗅诊的研究由于数据采集过程中环境干扰因素交错,大多仍关注于采集仪器的研制和数据去噪等质量提升工作方面,智能化的诊断还相对较少。当前研究热点中舌诊和面诊均是直接针对采集图像进行学习,早期多采用传统的图像处理技术,后来则逐渐采用机器学习的方法。切诊可看作是在二维脉图数据上通过信号处理或学习的方式完成分析与预测。问诊数据大多为量表化数据,在选择和推荐问诊问题时,大多数研究仍采用基于图模型、内容或领域的传统推荐算法。在针对获取到的问诊数据进行证候分类时则多采用机器学习或深度学习建模的方式来完成。与此同时,智能化四诊设备应运而生,并朝着小型化、移动化和可穿戴化发展,适用于日常生活的健康状态管理。

As a treasure of Chinese civilization, traditional Chinese medicine has played an important role and made great contributions in fighting against both SARS and COVID-19 epidemic.

Under the background of inheritance, development and innovation of traditional Chinese medicine, four diagnostic methods, as the basis of diagnosis and syndrome differentiation of traditional Chinese medicine, play a huge role in disease diagnosis and treatment. They are efficient and accurate.

Four diagnostic methods in traditional Chinese medicine include inspection, listening and smelling, inquire and palpation. They have been gradually formed and developed on the basis of the long-term medical practice of physicians in past dynasties, and have been supplemented and improved with the progress of the times. ①Inspection is the diagnostic method that doctors observe the abnormal changes in the whole body or local regions of the patients in order to understand the pathological conditions. It covers various aspects such as the vitality, spirit, complexion, posture, tongue and coating, excreta and index fingers of children. ②Listening and smelling is the diagnostic method to understand the pathological conditions by listening to the abnormal sounds and smelling the odors emitted from the patients. ③Inquiry is the diagnostic method to understand the occurrence and progression of disease, previous treatment, present subjective symptoms and other things concerning the disease by asking the patient or his or her companion. ④Palpation is the diagnostic method performed by pressing certain parts of the body. Physicians use fingers and palms to take the pulse, knock or press certain parts of the body, observe the reaction and physical conditions of the patients so that they can understand the pathological conditions and treat the disease.

1 Basic Contents of Four Diagnostic Methods

1.1 Basic Procedures and Methods

Four diagnostic methods are used to collect disease data from different perspectives. In practical application, the four methods should be given equal emphasis and doctors need to comprehensively analyse the data gained by four diagnostic methods.

In clinical application, doctors usually take inquiry first. During inquiry, they may use inspection, listening and smelling as well as palpation successively or interactively according to the specific situation of the patient to obtain disease data comprehensively.

To get the data which cannot be directly obtained by inspection or listening and smelling, doctors can ask the patient and his or her companion. Meanwhile, it's also possible to get the data when available afterwards.

1.2 Basic Requirements

In general, the four diagnostic operations should be carried out in a quiet, tidy and well-ventilated consulting room, where the temperature, humidity and air pressure are kept within a comfortable range, so that the sensitivity of the doctor's various senses is minimally affected.

The consulting room should be provided with articles and equipment needed for the operations, such as cushion, flashlight, tongue depressor. Pay attention to protecting patients' privacy when it requires them to expose their body.

The four diagnostic operations are best selected to be carried out during the day, and patients treated at night should recheck during the day if necessary.

1.3 Precautions

1.3.1 Psychosomatic State

Ensure that patients undergo examination in the state of calm, uniform breathing, relaxation and active cooperation.

When patients are unable to cooperate with some operations due to delirium and coma, language disorders and hearing disorders, or they are unwillingness to cooperate, physicians can adjust their operation flexibly according to actual situation and obtain the patient's information as much as possible.

1.3.2 Position

Patients are usually in a sitting or supine position. Doctors should guide patients to change their position or take corresponding actions to cooperate with the examination according to the needs of diagnosis.

According to the needs of inspection and palpation, patients should fully expose the tongue manifestation and pay attention to bilateral comparison.

When palpation, objects that may oppress the treated arm such as watches, shoulder bags and fastened cuffs need to be removed.

1.3.3 Dressing

Doctors should observe whether patients wear makeup, dye their hair, or wear artificial limbs and other auxiliary devices to correct their limbs. Distinguish changes caused by human factors.

1.3.4 Internal and External Environment

Doctors should pay attention to the influence of internal and external factors such as age, gender, physique, race, season, day and night, geographical environment, as well as drinking, diet, drugs, mood, exercise, sun and other factorson complexion, tongue manifestations and pulse condition.

1.4 Specific Operation of Four Diagnostic Methods

1.4.1 Inspection

During the short period of contact with the patient, the doctor should first observe the overall condition of the patient (such as spirit, complexion, physical build and movement). On this basis, according to the needs of disease diagnosis, observe the local conditions of the patient (such as head, face, neck, body, limbs, urino – genitals and anus, skin, etc.) and excretions (such as sputum, saliva, phlegm, vomitus, urine and feces). Under normal circumstances, the tongue manifestations of each patient should be observed.

For infants under 3 years old, doctors should also observe the superficial veins on index fingers.

When inspection, try to exclude the physiological changes (such as diet, temperature, emotions) caused by various internal and external factors and the changes caused by human factors (such as hair dyeing, makeup), compare the complexion changes of patients with the normal ones.

1.4.2 Listening and Smelling

Doctors should listen carefully to the voice and also smell the odors emitted from the patient when communicating with the patient or having physical examinations.

If the patient has symptoms of abnormal sound or smell but has no manifestation at that time, relevant data can be obtained by asking the patient and his or her companion.

1.4.3　Inquiry

In clinical practice,according to the specific situation of the patients,such as initial or follow-up consultation,acute or chronic diseases,doctors should make systematic,comprehensive and focused inquiries about the problems found during diagnosis and the problems related to the disease.

For patients with newly diagnosed chronic diseases,first ask the main complaint,then conduct detailed inquiries on the history of present illness and anamnesis. If necessary,ask about their family history and personal history.

For patients with acute or critical diseases,the physician should first determine the main symptoms through a brief interview with the patient or a companion and perform a focused examination to quickly treat or relieve the pain of the patient. After the illness is relieved or stabilized,doctors can ask for other contents related to theillness in detail.

For patients with repeated visits and have established medical records,doctors should first browse the past medical records to understand the anamnesis and present illness,and then ask about the reasons for this visit or the recent changes of the illness and therapeutic effects.

1.4.4　Palpation

(1) Breathing: Doctor should regulate and balance his own breathing pattern,calm and concentrate,calculate the number of pulse beats of the patient through his own breathing.

(2) Finger Positioning Method

1) Finger Positioning: The doctor uses the index finger,middle finger and ring finger of the left or right hand to diagnose the pulse.

First,the three fingertips should be aligned,presenting the shape of an arc. Then,to locate the *Guan* (medial aspect of the styloid process) position with the middle finger,the *Cun* (anterior to *Guan*) position with the index finger and the *Chi* (posterior to *Guan*) position with the ring finger. The fingers should be closely attached to the pulsating area at an angle of about 45 degrees to the patient's body surface.

Adjust the distances between the fingers according to the patients' height and arm length.

For patients with taller height and longer arms,the finger placement should be sparse,and vice versa.

2) Locating *Cunkou* position with One Finger: For children,doctors should use the thumb or the index finger to press the radial styloid pulse behind the palm. When diagnosing,use one finger to slide or move to both sides to feel the pulse of the three parts (*Cun*,*Guan* and *Chi*).

3) Operation Means: according to the order and specific conditions of patients,doctors can exert different finger pressures on positions for pulse examination and use different pulse diag-

nosis methods such as overall pulse examination, one finger pressing examination and locating *Cunkou with one finger to observe pulse conditions*.

(3) The Time of Pulse Examination: The time of pulse examination should be no less than 1 min for each hand, and it is appropriate to take a 3−min diagnosis for two hands to observe the change of pulse conditions.

2 Current Researches of Four Diagnostic Methods

As the basic methods of traditional Chinese medicine diagnosis, the four diagnostic methods are mainly applied to the diagnosis of various diseases and the identification of physique in clinic. However, the four diagnostic methods require doctors to analyze the data of patients and make accurate judgments based on experience. It's an extremely subjective form of diagnosis and has high requirements for doctors. Therefore, the objectification of four diagnostic methods in traditional Chinese medicine has become the development direction.

In recent years, with the rapid development of artificial intelligence technology, some scholars have used natural language processing, computer vision, knowledge graph, and deep learning to promote the development of four diagnostic methods in the direction of data, standardization, objectification and intelligence. Scholars have summarized the standardization and objectification of single method or the integration of four diagnostic methods from the aspects of historical development or clinical diagnostic technology.

At present, the hotspots of intelligent research on four diagnostic methods are mainly focused on tongue diagnosis, face diagnosis, palpation and inquiry.

Due to the interference of environmental factors in data collection, most of the researches on the diagnostic method of listening and smelling still focus on the development of collection instruments and quality improvement work such as data denoising. There is relatively little research on intelligent diagnosis.

In the current research hotspots, both tongue diagnosis and face diagnosis are focused on the collected images. In the early stage, they mostly use the traditional image processing technology, and then gradually adopt the method of machine learning.

Palpation can be regarded as the analysis and prediction of two−dimensional pulse map data by signal processing or learning. Most of the inquiry data are scale−based. When selecting and recommending the questions, most studies still adopt traditional recommendation algorithms based on graph model, content or field. Machine learning or deep learning modeling is often used to classify the syndromes from the collected information.

At the same time, intelligent four diagnostic devices emerged and have evolved toward miniaturization, mobility, and wear-ability, suitable for health state management in daily life.

第二节 辨证论治
(Treatment Based on Pattern Differentiation)

早在战国时期,《黄帝内经》就已经记载了许多中医证候的名称及其临床表现,为辨证论治体系的形成奠定了理论基础。至东汉时期,张仲景在《伤寒杂病论》中较为明确地提出了辨证论治的概念,并创立了比较完整的辨证论治体系。此后,历代医家又从不同角度大大丰富和发展了辨证论治的内容,形成了现有的辨证论治体系。

辨证论治,又称辨证施治,是理、法、方、药运用于临床的过程,是中医认识疾病和治疗疾病的基本原则。包括辨证和论治两个过程。所谓辨证,即通过四诊八纲、脏腑、病因、病机等中医基础理论对患者表现的症状、体征进行综合分析,辨别为何种病证。所谓论治,即结合临床经验,形成治则治法和治疗方案,并通过反馈调整治疗方案最终达到防治疾病目的的过程。

一、辨证论治主要内容(Main Contents of Treatment Based on Pattern Differentiation)

在中医学发展过程中,历代医家针对各类疾病的不同特点,创立了多种辨证方法。这些辨证方法各具特点,又互有联系,体现了相应的辨证内容。

（一）八纲辨证

八纲辨证是中医基本辨证纲领之一。它是在收集各种临床资料的基础上对病变部位、证候的性质、正气的盛衰、邪气的强弱,以及病证的发展趋势等所做出的阴、阳、表、里、寒、热、虚、实八类证候的诊断归纳。其中表和里表示病位的浅深,寒和热概括证候的性质,虚和实表现正邪的盛衰,而阴和阳是对表、里、寒、热、虚、实的高度概括,即表证、热证、实证可归属为阳证;里证、寒证、虚证归属为阴证。以上八类证候常错综夹杂,相兼出现,如表寒证、里热证、虚寒证等。八纲的四对矛盾,是相对的,互相联系、互相转化的。临床上错综复杂的证候都可以用它作分析归纳的基本方法。

（二）脏腑辨证

脏腑辨证是以脏腑的生理功能和病理特点为理论依据,来判断病变属何脏、何腑及其气血阴阳虚实寒热等变化,从而为治疗提供依据的辨证方法。如脾主运化水谷精微,为气血生化之源,因而临床见有纳少、腹胀、便溏、肢倦、少气懒言、面色萎黄者,即可辨为脾气虚证。由于这种辨证方法将病变部位落实到具体脏腑,因而其辨证层次较深入,针对性较强。脏腑辨证是临床各科的辨证基础,是辨证体系中的重要组成部分。

（三）病因辨证

运用中医病因病机理论,对四诊所得的临床资料进行综合分析,以推求判断疾病的发病原因,为治疗提供依据的辨证方法。病因辨证的关键,是根据各种病因的致病特点,分析患者的临床表现,推求判断病因种类而对证治疗。病因包括六淫（风、寒、暑、湿、燥、火）、疫疬（疠气、毒气、异气、戾气、杂气、瘟疫）、七情（喜、怒、忧、思、悲、恐、惊）、痰、瘀、食、虫等致病因素。

（四）气血辨证

运用藏象学说中有关气血的理论,分析各种临床表现,从而判断气、血方面病变的一种辨证方法。例如,血有营养和滋润全身脏腑组织的生理功能,若见面白无华或萎黄,唇色淡白,爪甲苍白,头晕眼花,心悸失眠,妇女月经不调,即可辨为血虚证。由于气血既是脏腑功能活动的物质基础,又是脏腑功能活动的产物,因而气血病变与脏腑病变密切相关,气血辨证与脏腑辨证常需结合运用。

（五）经络辨证

根据十二经脉、奇经八脉循行部位及其相关脏腑的功能特点,分析疾病时的临床表现,从而判断病变所属经脉的一种辨证方法。如手太阴肺经病证,可见咳喘,胸部满闷,手臂内侧前缘疼痛等。经脉联络脏腑,运行气血,其病变相互影响,因而经络辨证应与脏腑辨证、气血辨证参合运用。

（六）六经辨证

根据外感病（指感受六淫等外邪而引起的疾病）发生、发展、变化的一般规律及其临床表现特点,以太阳、阳明、少阳、太阴、少阴、厥阴六经作为辨证纲领,对外感病演变过程中所表现的各种证候,从正气的强弱、病邪的盛衰、病情的进退缓急等方面,进行分析、归纳、综合,找出其固有的发展规律和内在联系,为治疗提供依据。六经辨证中包含有八纲、脏腑、气血津液、经络、病因等辨证方法的内容,它们之间具有密切的内在联系。

（七）三焦辨证

根据温病发生发展的一般规律及症状变化的特点,以上焦、中焦、下焦为辨证纲领,对温病发展过程中的各种临床表现进行综合分析和概括,用以判断病理阶段,归纳证候类型,明确病变部位,确立治疗原则,并借以推测预后转归。

在辨证基础上即可论治,确立治疗原则,选择治疗方法,并确定处方用药。疾病的证候表现多种多样,病理变化极为复杂,病变有轻重缓急,不同的时间、地点以及不同的个体都会对病情变化产生不同影响。通过辨证,分清疾病的现象和本质,即可求本治疗;辨清邪正斗争的虚实变化,即可扶正祛邪;根据阴阳失调的病理变化,予以调整阴阳;按脏腑、气血失调的病机,予以调整脏腑功能,调整气血关系;按发病的不同时间、地点和患者的不同个体特点,予以因时、因地、因人制宜的治疗。在上述原则的指导下,根据不同的病因、病位、病性、病机就可确定具体的治疗方法,进而选择有效的方药。

二、辨证论治发展现状（Current Researches of Treatment Based on Pattern Differentiation）

辨证论治以阴阳、五行、脏腑、经络、气血津液、病因病机、治则等中医基本理论为依据,通过理法方药的表现形式,使中医理论体系在临床实践中得到应用。关于辨证论治的概念,在中医学界有不同的理解。有人将方剂辨证纳入辨证论治范围,即某一方剂常有一定的适应证,通过辨别不同方剂的对应证候,可为选用方剂提供依据。近年来随着控制论、系统论、信息论等新学科向中医领域的渗透,有人认为辨证论治是医生收集患者信息,进行信息的提取、分析和对问题进行处理的过程。辨证就是对信息的提取和分析,找出疾病函数或相关的特征值;论治就是输出治疗信息,排除干扰,实现校正的过程。从数学上看,辨证论治包括模糊数学、集合论和映射论等概念;有人根据对泛系理论的研究,提出辨证论治在本质上可以通过聚类、模拟、观控和判别的泛系模式来形成多种数学模型。电子计算机在辨证论治中得到较广泛的应用,计算机专家系统、人工智能和辅助诊断在一定程度上反映了辨证论治的思维方式,这有利于辨证论治向规范化、标准化、检测化发展。

根据现代研究,辨证论治还有不完善之处。由于辨证论治中存在许多不确定的因素,定量性可检测的参数较少,因而具有一定的不清晰性和随机性,易受假象干扰和主观因素的影响。辨证论治缺乏对微观层次的认识。对某些虽有器质性病变,但因代偿而处于尚未表现功能异常的隐匿状态的疾病,或者临床症状消失,但内脏器官组织尚存病变的状态尚难认识,诊断和治疗手段存在局限。另外,辨证论治中的一些名词概念尚不统一或不规范,在法律诊断、劳动力鉴定上缺乏明确标准。这些因素使辨证论治的运用受到一定限制,与当代医疗的需要有不相适应之处。近年来,中医学界对辨证论治理论的规范化和系统的完整化,辨证论治的方法和步骤等问题,做了不少探讨,正致力于建立辨证论治的新体系。

As early as the Warring States Period, *Huangdi Neijing*(*Yellow Emperor's Canon of Medicine*) already recorded many names of TCM patterns and their clinical manifestations, laying a theoretical foundation for the formation of treatment based on pattern differentiation system.

Up to the Eastern Han Dynasty, Zhang Zhongjing clearly put forward the concept of treatment based on pattern differentiation in *Shanghan Zabing Lun* (*Treatise on Cold Pathogenic and Miscellaneous Diseases*), and established a relatively complete system of treatment based on pattern differentiation.

Since then, physicians in different dynasties have greatly enriched and developed the content of treatment based on pattern differentiation, forming the existing system.

Treatment based on pattern differentiation is the clinical process in which theory, method, prescription and medicinal are applied. It's a basic principle in TCM for understanding and treating diseases, which includes two processes: pattern differentiation and treatment.

Pattern differentiation is to comprehensively analyze the symptoms and signs of patients through the basic theories of traditional Chinese medicine such as four diagnostic methods, eight principles, *zang-fu* organs, etiology, and pathogenesis to identify what kind of pattern it is.

Treatment is the process of combining clinical experience to form a therapeutic rule and a treatment plan, and adjusting the treatment plan through feedback to finally achieve the purpose of preventing and treating diseases.

1 Main Contents of Treatment Based on Pattern Differentiation

In the development of traditional Chinese medicine, physicians of all ages have established a variety of pattern differentiation methods according to different characteristics of various diseases.

These methods have their own characteristics and are related to each other, which reflect the corresponding contents.

1.1 Pattern Differentiation of Eight Principles

Pattern differentiation of eight principles is one of the basic principles of TCM syndrome differentiation. On the basis of collecting all kinds of clinical data, it differentiates diseases into *yin*, *yang*, exterior, interior, cold, heat, deficiency and excess patterns through analysing the data on the disease location, nature, strength between healthy *qi* and pathogenic *qi*, and the development trend of patterns.

Among these patterns, exterior and interior indicate the location of disease, cold and heat generalize the nature of syndrome, deficiency and excess show waxing and waning of healthy *qi* and pathogenic factors, while *yin* and *yang* highly generalize the characteristics of those six patterns.

That is, exterior pattern, heat pattern and excess pattern can be classified as *yang* pattern, while interior pattern, cold pattern and deficiency pattern belong to *yin* pattern.

The above eight kinds of patterns are often intermingle and concurrent, manifesting as exterior cold pattern, interior heat pattern and deficiency cold pattern, etc. The four pairs of contradictions of the eight principles are relative, interconnected and mutually transformed. They can be used as a basic method for analysis and induction of complex patterns in clinic.

1.2 Pattern Differentiation of *Zang-Fu* Organs

Pattern differentiation of *zang-fu* organs is a diagnosis and treatment method. Based on the physiological function and pathological characteristics of *zang-fu* organs, it can deduce the disease location and judge the pathological changes such as *qi*, blood, *yin*, *yang*, deficiency, excess, cold and heat, so as to provide basis for treatment.

For example, the spleen transports and transforms the grain essence, it is considered as the source of *qi* and blood. In clinical, the spleen deficiency pattern can be distinguished from poor appetite, abdominal distension, urination, lassitude, lack of energy, no desire to speak and yellowish complexion.

Since this method studies the lesion part of the specific viscera, it has strong pertinence compared with other methods. It's the basis of pattern differentiation in clinical and an important part of syndrome differentiation system.

1.3 Pattern Differentiation of Etiology

Pattern differentiation of etiology is a method of diagnosis and treatment. By using the theory of etiology and pathogenesis of traditional Chinese medicine, it comprehensively analyzes the clinical data collected by the four diagnostic methods, judges the causes of diseases, and provides a basis for disease treatment.

The key to pattern differentiation of etiology is to analyze the clinical manifestations of patients, judge the types of etiology and treat the syndrome according to the pathogenic characteristics of various causes.

Etiology, refers to the factors that result in disease, including six excesses (wind, cold, summer heat, dampness, dryness and fire), pestilence, seven emotions (joy, anger, anxiety, thought, sorrow, fear and fright), phlegm, stasis of blood, improper diet, insect or animal bites, etc.

1.4 Pattern Differentiation of *Qi* and Blood

Pattern differentiation of *qi* and blood is a method to analyse clinical pathologies of *qi* and blood according to the relevant theories of the *zang-fu* organs.

For example, blood has the physiological function of nourishing and moistening all the organs and tissues of the whole body. Therefore, blood deficiency pattern can be manifested as pale or sallow facial complexion, pale lips, pale nails, dizziness, palpitation, insomnia, and menstrual disorders.

Since *qi* and blood are the material basis and the products of functional activities of *zang-fu* organs, the pathological changes of *qi* and blood are closely related to the pathological changes of *zang-fu* organs, these two pattern differentiation methods often need to be used in combination.

1.5 Pattern Differentiation of Meridians

Pattern differentiation of meridians is a method to analyse clinical signs of disease, identify the specific meridians according to the circulation positions of twelve meridians and eight extra meridians as well as the functional characteristics of related *zang-fu* organs.

For example, lung meridian pattern is characterized by cough, asthma, chest distress and fullness, as well as pain in the ulnar anterior border of the arm.

The meridians are pathways in which the *qi* and blood of the human body are circulated. They link the tissues and organs into an organic whole. Since the pathological changes of meridians, *qi* and blood as well as *zang-fu* organs influence each other, these three pattern differentiation methods should be used in combination.

1.6 Pattern Differentiation of Six Meridians

Pattern differentiation of six meridians is a method that provides a basis for treatment by analyzing the general rules and clinical characteristics of the externally contracted disorders (a group of disorders caused by external pathogenic factors such as six excesses) in the aspect of symptoms, strength between healthy *qi* and pathogenic factors, and the development trend of patterns. The six meridians refer to *Taiyang* meridian, *Yangming* meridian, *Shaoyang* meridian, *Taiyin* meridian, *Shaoyin* meridian and *Jueyin* meridian. The content of pattern differentiation of six meridians includes eight principles, *zang-fu* organs, *qi*, blood and body fluids, meridians, etiology and other pattern differentiation methods. There is a close internal relationship among them.

1.7 Pattern Differentiation of *Sanjiao*

Pattern differentiation of the three *jiao* is a method of diagnosis and treatment. Based on the three transmission stages (upper *jiao*, middle *jiao* and lower *jiao*) of febrile diseases, through comprehensive analysis of clinical manifestations and symptom changes of febrile diseases, this method can judge the pathological stage, summarize the syndrome types, clarify the lesion location, and finally establish the treatment principles. It can also be used for prognosis.

On the basis of pattern differentiation, we can discuss the treatment of diseases, establish the treatment principles, choose the treatment method, and determine the prescriptions.

The patterns of diseases are varied, the pathological changes are extremely complex, and the lesions have priorities. Time, place, physical condition and other factors will have different effects on the changes of diseases.

Through pattern differentiation, the phenomenon and essence of the disease can be distinguished, and then the treatment can be carried out according to the main etiology of the disease.

By distinguishing the deficiency and excess changes of healthy *qi* and pathogenic factors, we can reinforce healthy *qi* to eliminate pathogenic factors.

By analyzing the pathological changes of disharmony between *yin* and *yang*, we can harmonize *yin* and *yang*.

According to the pathogenesis of *zang-fu* organs and *qi*-blood imbalance, we can adjust the function of *zang-fu* organs and the relationship between *qi* and blood.

Because of the time, place and the characteristics of patients are different, doctors should give treatment according to time, place and person.

Under the guidance of the above principles, specific treatment methods can be determined according to the cause, location, nature and pathogenesis of diseases. Then, effective prescriptions can be selected.

2　Current Researches of Treatment Based on Pattern Differentiation

Treatment based on pattern differentiation developed the basic theories of traditional Chinese medicine, such as *yin-yang*, five-elements, *zang-fu* organs, meridians, *qi*, blood and body fluids, etiology and etiology, as well as the principles of treatment. Through the manifestations of theory, principle, prescription and medicinal, the theoretical system of TCM has been applied in clinical practice.

There are different understandings about the concept of treatment based on pattern differentiation in TCM.

Some bring prescription differentiation into the scope of treatment based on pattern differentiation. That is, a prescription often has certain indications, by identifying the corresponding syndromes of different prescriptions, it can provide a basis for the selection of prescriptions.

In recent years, with the penetration of new disciplines such as cybernetics, system theory and information theory into the field of traditional Chinese medicine, some people consider treatment based on pattern differentiation as a process in which doctors collect the data of patients, extract and analyze the data and then treat the diseases.

Pattern differentiation is to extract and analyze the data and find out disease function or related eigenvalues.

Treatment is the process of outputting treatment information, eliminating interference and realizing correction.

From a mathematical point of view, treatment based on pattern differentiation includes the concepts of fuzzy mathematics, set theory and mapping theory.

According to the study of pan-system theory, it is proposed that treatment based on pattern differentiation can essentially form a variety of mathematical models through the pan-system model of clustering, simulation, observation, control and discrimination.

Computer has been widely used in treatment based on pattern differentiation. The computer expert system, artificial intelligence and auxiliary diagnosis reflect the thinking mode of this method to a certain extent, which is conducive to the development of it towards standardization, standardization and detection.

According to modern researches, there are still imperfections in treatment based on pattern differentiation.

There are many uncertain factors and few quantitative detectable parameters in treatment based on pattern differentiation. So it has a certain degree of ambiguity and randomness, which is easily disturbed by illusions and is easily affected by subjective factors.

It lacks the understanding of the micro level.

There are limitations in diagnosis and treatment. For example, it is difficult to diagnose some diseases which have organic lesions but are in a hidden state without abnormal function due to compensation. Also, it is difficult to recognize the condition in which the clinical symptoms disappear but the internal organ tissue remains diseased.

In addition, some concepts in treatment based on pattern differentiation are not uniformed or standardized. There are no clear standards in legal diagnosis and labor force appraisal.

These factors restrict the application of treatment based on pattern differentiation to a certain extent, which is inconsistent with the needs of contemporary medical treatment.

In recent years, TCM scholars have made a lot of discussions on the standardization, systematization, methods and steps of the treatment based on pattern differentiation theory. They are devoting themselves to establishing a new system of it.

第三节 天人合一
(Unity of Human and Nature)

2017 年 1 月 19 日,国家主席习近平在出席"共商共筑人类命运共同体"高级别会议发表主旨演讲时指出:"我们应该遵循天人合一、道法自然的理念,寻求永续发展之路。""天人合一"思想作为"和合"理念的重要组成部分,在中华优秀传统文化中具有独特内涵与意义。在《黄帝内经》开篇处,有言:"阴阳者,天地之道也,万物之纲纪,变化之父母,生杀之本始,神明之府也。"从宇宙论层面讲述了万物生成消亡皆是阴阳所决定的,又以五行学说将阴阳推向了属于具体事物的五行维度,为构建阴阳、精气、五味、五方、五脏为主的"天人合一"的中医学整体观打下基础。

天人合一,是指天、地、人本原于一气,同构同律,相参相应的思维方式。天,即天地、自然。天人合一属于古代哲学的命题之一,天、地、人关系密切,故可从天地的本质与现象来分析人的生命活动的规律。

一、天人合一主要内容（Main Contents of Unity of Human and Nature）

天人合一作为中医学的系统思维方式,指导着对人体生理、病理的认识,融汇在疾病的诊断和治疗措施中,因此,中医学始终把人的生命活动,放在天文地理、季节气候、民族民风、社会地位、社会责任、生活习惯等天、地、人三大要素构成的框架中去分析,以探寻本质和规律,预测其发展变化。

（一）天人同气

天人同气,即天、地、人同源于一气,"气"是包括人体生命在内的万事万物的本原。在天地未形成之前,这种运动不息的物质之气,便充满着整个太虚。人身之精气和自然界中的精气是同一种东西。人体生命和宇宙自然就是靠"气"构成了一个整体。天食人以五气,地食人以五味,从而维持人的生命活动。人与万物相同,生于天地气交之中,气质升降出入、聚散阖辟的运动变化,形成万物生长化收藏,人体生命活动的生长壮老已。

（二）天地同构

天地同构,即天、地、人的结构特征相同。"天人同构"是"天人合一"的空间结构层面。《黄帝内经》把人体形态结构与天地万物一一对应起来,人体的结构可以在自然界中找到相对应的东西,人体仿佛是天地的缩影。这就强调人的存在与自然存在是统一的。人身小宇宙,宇宙大人身。

（三）天人同律

天人同律,即天、地、人的节律相同。天地自然的节律主要为年、月、日、时,人亦应之。年节律,由于阴阳消长而形成春、夏、秋、冬季节更替,人以五脏系统相应,形成"四时五脏阴阳"整体观。月节律,由于月之朔望,形成大地海水潮汐节律变化,人之气血,月满则盈,月亏则虚。日节律,一日对应四季,日出为春,中午为夏,日落为秋,夜半为冬,并以此形成"子午流注"理论,应用于说明脏腑经络气血的生理功能、经病诊治、针灸按时取穴以及养生保健。

二、天人合一发展现状（Current Researches of Unity of Human and Nature）

天人合一作为中医学的主要思维方式之一,指导着医生对临床疾病进行诊断与治疗,如采用因人制宜、因时制宜、因地制宜的方法分析疾病发生发展规律,从而达到治疗效果,由此形成了时序发病观、音乐治疗观等观念。近年来,天人合一思维也广泛应用于中医养生相关领域,衍生出相关养生观念。顺应天时养生观:以四时二十四节为规律,五脏阴阳为根本,调整人体生命活动与自然界变化的周期同步,保持机体内外环境的协调统一。因人制宜养生观:个体的体质与健康和疾病的发生有着密不可分的关系,对不同人群体质的差异性,养生方法也要"因人制宜",找到个人适合的情况进行。未病先防、既病防变养生观:防病是养生的主要目的之一,而养生又是防病最有效的手段。中医治未病的思想充分体现了古人对疾病的预防观,即通过合理的治疗方法,来防止疾病的发生或发展。"形神共养"养生观:形神是人的一体两面,神有赖形而存在,形是神的依附,而神是形的主宰。"形神共养"养生观是中医养生的最高境界,也是中医养生学推崇的一种最高养生方法。

一些学者寻根溯源,深度解析《黄帝内经》中的天人合一思维,探究其对中医学的影响,也有学者提出随着社会的不断发展,人类所处的环境、已经从事的活动已发生了巨大的改变,因此,天人合一思维要与时俱进,拓宽、加入现代内涵。

In his keynote speech at the high-level meeting on "Building a Community with a Shared Future for Mankind" on Jan 19, 2017, General Secretary Xi Jinping pointed out: "We should follow the concept of unity of human and nature and the law of nature, try to seek a path of sustainable development."

As an important part of the vision of peace and harmony, the thought of "unity of human and nature" has a unique connotation and significance in excellent Chinese traditional culture.

At the beginning of *Huangdi Neijing* (*Yellow Emperor's Canon of Medicine*), there is a saying: "*Yin* and *yang* serve as the law of the heavens and the earth, the fundamental principle of all things, the parents of change, the beginning of birth and death and the storehouse of *Shenming* (spirit). "

From the perspective of cosmology, it tells that the generation, growth, collapse and death of all things are determined by *yin* and *yang*. The theory of five-elements pushes *yin* and *yang* to the five-elements dimension belonging to specific things, laying the foundation for the construction of the holistic view "unity of human and nature" in traditional Chinese medicine, which is based on *yin* and *yang*, essence, five flavors, five directions and five *zang*-organs.

Unity of human and nature refers to the thinking mode that the heaven, the earth and human are all originated from *qi*, and they are related to each other.

Heaven also refers to the earth and nature.

Unity of human and nature is one of the propositions of ancient philosophy. Since heaven, the earth and human are closely related, the nature and phenomenon of heaven and earth can be used to analyze the law of human activities.

1　Main Contents of Unity of Human and Nature

As a systematic thinking mode of traditional Chinese medicine, unity of human and nature guides the understanding of human physiology and pathology, and integrates into the diagnosis and treatment of diseases. Therefore, traditional Chinese medicine always analyzes people's life activities in the framework of the three elements such as astronomy, geography, seasonal climate, ethnic customs, socialstatus, social responsibility and living habits, explores the essence and laws of human and nature, and then predicts their development and changes.

1.1　Human and Nature Sharing the Same Origin

Human and nature share the same origin. The heaven, the earth and human all originate from *qi*, which is the origin of all things including human life. Before the formation of the heaven and the earth, the whole universe was full of this kind of moving *qi*.

The essence *qi* of human body is the same thing as the essence *qi* of nature. Human life and the universe form a whole through "*qi*".

The heaven provides man with five kinds of *qi* and the earth provides man with five kinds of flavors, thus maintaining people's life activities. Human and things in the universe are all born in the intersection of *qi*. The movement and change of *qi* (such as ascending, descending, entering and exiting, gathering and dispersing) is the condition for human life activities and the growth and extinction of all things.

1.2　Human and Nature Sharing the Same Structure

The structural characteristics of the heaven, the earth and human are the same. It's the space structure level of unity of human and nature.

In *Huangdi Neijing* (*Yellow Emperor's Canon of Medicine*), it corresponds the structure of the human body to all things in the universe. The structure of the human body can find the corresponding things in nature, and the human body seems to be the epitome of the heaven and the earth. This is to emphasize that human and natural coexist in harmony. The human body is like a small universe, while the universe is a large human body.

1.3　Human and Nature Sharing the Same Law

The law of the heaven, the earth and human is the same. The rhythms of the heaven and the earth are the year, month, day and hour, and people should also follow them.

The rule of the year refers to the change of four seasons due to the waxing and waning between *yin* and *yang*. The system of five *zang*-organs corresponds to it, forming a holistic view of the "four seasons, five organs and *yin—yang*".

The rule of the luna refers to the changes of the earth, sea and tides due to the lunar solstices. Corresponding to this, the *qi* and blood of human body are full when the moon is full and deficient when the moon is wane.

The rule of the solar corresponds to the four seasons: sunrise for spring, noon for summer, sunset for autumn, and midnight for winter. The theory of "Midnight—noon ebb—flow" is formed based on it, which is applied to explain the physiological functions of *zang—fu* organs, meridians, *qi* and blood. It is also applied to the diagnosis and treatment of meridian diseases, acupuncture and health care.

2   Current Researches of Unity of Human and Nature

As one of the main thinking modes of traditional Chinese medicine, the concept of unity of human and nature guides doctors to diagnose and treat clinical diseases. Under this thinking mode, doctors adopt the methods to treat according to person, time and place so as to achieve therapeutic effects, thus forming concepts such as time sequence and music therapy.

In recent years, this thinking mode has also been widely used in the fields related to health preservation in traditional Chinese medicine, deriving the related views on health preservation.

Health preservation in accordance with the times: It takes the four seasons and twenty—four solar terms as the rules and the five *zang* organs and *yin—yang* as the fundamentals to adjust the human body's life activities. Synchronize the life activities of the human body with the cycles of nature and maintain the harmony of the internal and external environment of the body.

Health preservation in accordance with personal conditions: There is a close relationship between the physical constitution of individual and the occurrence of diseases. For people with different physiques, there are different methods of health preservation, and one should find a method suitable for themselves.

Preventing a disease before it arises and preventing transmission of a disease after its onset: Disease prevention is one of the main purposes of health preservation, and in turn, health preservation is the most effective means of disease prevention.

The idea of preventing a disease before it arises in TCM fully reflects the ancients' thoughts of disease prevention. That is, to prevent a disease before it arises and prevent transmission of a disease after its onset.

Preserving both the body and the mind: Body and mind are the two sides of human beings, the existence of the mind depends on the body, and the mind is the master of the body.

The concept of "preserving both the body and the mind" is the highest state of traditional

Chinese medicine health preservation, and it is also the most respected method of health preservation in traditional Chinese medicine.

Some scholars have traced their roots and deeply analyzed the idea of unity of human and nature in *Huangdi Neijing* (*Yellow Emperor's Canon of Medicine*) and explored its influence on traditional Chinese medicine while others have suggested that with the development of society, the environment has changed dramatically. Therefore, the idea should keep pace with the times, and add the modern connotations.

第四节　阴阳学说
(*Yin-Yang* Theory)

阴阳学说对于中医学而言,是有着极为特殊的意义与地位的,其贯穿于中医学理论体系的各个层面,既是中医学构建理论体系所必需的核心观念与基本指导思想,又是中医学进行医疗实践和理论研究的重要理论工具,同时也参与藏象、经络、病机、治疗、方药、针灸、养生等中医理论的主要内容组成,此外还是中医学与中国传统文化相互联系的具体体现。

阴阳的概念,属于中国古代哲学范畴,是对相关事物或同一事物本身存在的对立双方属性的概括,既可表示相关联又相对应的两种事物或现象的属性划分及运动变化,又可表示同一事物内部相互对应着的两个方面的属性趋向及运动规律。

中医学关于阴阳基本概念的经典表述,见于《素问·阴阳应象大论》:"阴阳者,天地之道也,万物之纲纪,变化之父母,生杀之本始,神明之府也。"阴阳是自然界的法则和规律,世界万物运动变化的纲领和根本,贯穿事物新生消亡的始终,是事物发生、发展和变化的内在动力。

一、阴阳学说主要内容(Main Contents of *Yin-Yang* Theory)

阴阳学说是以阴阳的对立统一及其相互作用阐释宇宙间万物的生成、发展和变化的根本规律,其主要内容包括阴阳交感、阴阳对立、阴阳互根、阴阳消长、阴阳转化、阴阳自和等方面。

(一)阴阳交感

阴阳交感,指阴阳二气在运动中相互感应而交合的相互作用。阴阳交通相合,彼此交感相错,是宇宙万物赖以生成和变化的根源。阴阳交感是天地万物化生的基础。阳气升腾而为天,阴气凝聚而为地。天气下降,地气上升,天地阴阳二气相互作用,交感合和,产生万物。在自然界,天地阴阳二气交感,形成云、雾、雷电、雨露,万物得以化生。人类作为宇宙万物之一,同样由天地阴阳之气交感合和而生成。生命便是在天地阴阳交互作用下孕育生息。如果没有阴阳二气的交感运动,就没有自然界万物,也就没有生命。

阴阳交感是事物和现象发展变化的动力。阴和阳属性相反,两者不断相摩相荡,发生交互作用,宇宙万物才能生生不息,变化无穷。

(二)阴阳对立

对立是指处于一个统一体的矛盾双方互相排斥、互相斗争。阴阳对立是阴阳双方的互相排斥、互相斗争。阴阳学说认为,对立相反是阴阳的基本属性,宇宙间很多事物和现象都存在对立相反的两个方面。如天与地、日与月、水与火、男与女、寒与热、动与静、上与下、左与右等。

阴阳对立的形式,通过阴阳之间的相互斗争、相互制约而发挥作用。阴可制约阳,阳能制约阴。阴阳相互制约是自然界四时寒暑往复变化的根源。人体正常生理活动具有兴奋和抑制的两种状态,即兴奋为阳,抑制属阴,彼此相互制约。昼则阳制约阴,人处于兴奋清醒状态;夜则阴制约阳,进入安静睡眠状态。阴阳对立相反而有昼夜寤寐的不同变化,动静相制维持人体寤和寐的正常节律,充分体现了阴阳双方的相互对立、相互制约。

阴阳对立的意义,在于防止阴阳的任何一方不至于亢盛为害,以维持阴阳之间的协调平衡。阴阳双方始终处于矛盾运动之中,在一定的限度内,由于阴阳双方相互斗争和相互制约的作用,才能够使阴阳的任何一方既无太过,也无不及,从而实现事物或现象内部及其相互之间的动态平衡,才能生生不息。如果阴阳双方中的一方过亢,对另一方制约太过;或阴阳双方中的一方不及,不能制约对方,则阴阳之间的对立制约关系失调,彼此之间的动态平衡被破坏,则会导致疾病发生。

(三)阴阳互根

阴阳互根,指相互对立的阴阳两个方面,具有相辅相成、相互依存的关系。阴阳互根的形式,通过阴阳互藏、互为根本而发挥作用。

阴阳互藏,指相互对立的阴阳双方中的任何一方都包含着另一方,即阴中有阳,阳中有阴。宇宙中的任何事物都含有阴与阳两种属性不同的成分,属阳的事物含有阴性成分,属阴的事物也寓有属阳的成分。以天地而言,天为阳,地为阴。天为地气升腾所形成,阳中蕴涵有阴;地乃天气下降所形成,则阴中蕴涵有阳。

阴阳互为根本,"阳根于阴,阴根于阳"。阳的根本在阴,阴的根本在阳,双方互为存在的前提。互为根本的阴阳双方具有相互资生、促进和助长的作用。

阴阳互藏互根的意义,在于阴阳始终处于统一体之中,每一方都以对方的存在作为自身存在的前提和条件,任何一方都不能脱离对方而单独存在。例如,春夏为阳,秋冬为阴,没有春夏,就无所谓秋冬;没有秋冬,就无所谓春夏。寒为阴,热为阳,没有寒,就无所谓热;反之亦然。阴不可无阳,阳不可无阴,阴阳双方密不可分。

（四）阴阳消长

阴阳消长,指阴阳双方不是静止不变的,而是处于不断地消减和增加的运动变化之中。消,减少、减退;长,增加、增长。古代哲学家认为,阴阳双方始终处于运动变化中,阴长阳消,阳长阴消。阴阳双方彼此的消减与增加的变化在一定的范围、限度、时空之内,保持着动态平衡。正是由于阴阳的消长变化,自然万物才能够维持相对、动态的平衡。

阴阳消长的形式,属于量变过程中进退、增减、盛衰的运动变化,包括此长彼消、此消彼长的阴阳互为消长与此长彼长、此消彼消的阴阳同消同长。

1. 阴阳互为消长　相互对立的阴阳双方,在彼此相互制约的过程中表现出互为消长的变化。表现形式有二:一是此长彼消,指阴或阳某一方增加而另一方随之出现消减的变化,即阳长阴消,阴长阳消。二是此消彼长,是阴或阳某一方消减而另一方随之出现增加的变化,即阳消阴长,阴消阳长。由于阴阳相互制约,阳长制约阴则阴消,阴长制约阳而阳消;若阳消而对阴的制约减弱则阴长,阴消对阳制约减弱则阳长。故阴阳互为消长是阴阳对立制约关系表现出的运动变化,而阴阳相互制约又在互为消长过程中实现。

自然界四时气候及昼夜的往复变化即是阴阳消长变化的体现,如一年四季的气候变化。人体生理活动也是阴阳消长的体现,子时一阳生,午时一阴生,人体的生理功能也由兴奋逐渐转向抑制,即"阴长阳消"的过程。

2. 阴阳同消同长　相互依存的阴阳双方,在彼此相互资助和促进的过程中表现出同消同长的变化。表现形式有二:一是此长彼长,是阴阳之间出现某一方增加而另一方亦增加,即阴随阳长或阳随阴长;二是此消彼消,是阴与阳之间出现某一方消减而另一方亦消减,即阴随阳消或阳随阴消。由于阴阳互为用,阳生可促进阴的化生;阴长又资助阳的生成;若阳消则阴无以化,阴消则阳无以生。阴阳同消同长是阴阳相互依存关系表现出的运动变化,而阴阳相互依存又在消长过程中实现。

四季气候变化,随着春夏气温的逐渐升高降雨量逐渐增多,随着秋冬气候的转凉而降雨量逐渐减少,即是阴阳同长与同消的消长变化。人体生理活动中,饥饿时出现的气力不足,即是由于精(阴)不足不能化生气(阳),属阳随阴消;而补充精(阴),产生能量(阳),增加了气力,则属阳随阴长。

阴阳消长的意义,在于维持阴阳双方相对的、动态的平衡状态。在一定的限度内,阴阳消长的运动变化,属于正常状态。例如,自然界的寒热温凉、人身的气血阴阳始终处在阴阳消长不断的运动变化之中,消而不偏衰,长而不偏亢,维持在一定范围之内,保持相对的动态平衡。自然界体现在正常气候变化,人体则体现在正常的生命活动。因此,阴阳消长是绝对的,阴阳平衡是相对的,保持阴阳双方在消长运动过程中的动态平衡极其重要。

（五）阴阳转化

阴阳转化，指事物的阴阳属性，在一定条件下可以向其相反的方向转化，即属阳的事物可以转化为属阴的事物，属阴的事物可以转化为属阳的事物。阴阳相互转化，一般都产生于事物发展变化的"物极"阶段，即所谓"物极必反"。当阴阳消长运动发展到一定阶段，"极则生变"，事物内部阴与阳的比例出现了颠倒，则该事物的属性即发生转化。

阴阳消长和转化都是阴阳运动变化的表现形式，但本质不同：阴阳消长是一个量变的过程，事物本身属性并未发生改变；阴阳转化是在量变基础上的质变，事物本身的属性转化为相反一面。阴阳转化是阴阳消长的结果。阴阳消长变化发展到"极"期是转化的条件，阴阳双方的消长运动发展超过一定的限度，则该事物的属性会发生转化。

（六）阴阳自和

阴阳自和，指阴阳双方自动维持和自动恢复其协调稳定状态的能力和趋势。阴阳自和是阴阳的本性。阴阳自和是以"自"为核心，依靠内在自我的相互作用而实现"和"。阴阳自和的机制，在于阴阳双方彼此的交互作用。阴阳虽然属性相反，但两者存在互生、互化、互制、互用等关系，在交互作用的变化中相反相成，是维持事物或现象协调发展的内在机制。

阴阳自和是相对的、动态的平衡，阴阳双方在交互作用中处于大体均势的状态，即阴阳协调和相对稳定状态。阴阳双方以对立制约与互根互用为基础，在一定限度内消长和在一定条件下转化的运动变化，维持阴阳平衡状态。

二、阴阳学说应用与发展现状（Current Researches of the Application and Development of *Yin–Yang* Theory）

中医学运用阴阳学说，以辩证思维指导对具体事物的认识，阐明生命的形体结构、功能活动、病机变化、临床诊断、疾病防治以及养生康复等，奠定了中医学理论体系的基础。

在阐释人体疾病变化方面，疾病的发生标志着阴阳协调关系的失衡，称为"阴阳失调"。中医学根据致病因素的性质及致病特点，把病因分为阴、阳两大类，如《素问·调经论》说："夫邪之生也，或生于阴，或生于阳。"一般而言，六淫属阳邪，情志失调、饮食居处等属阴邪。阴阳之中复有阴阳，如六淫之中，风邪、暑邪、火（热）邪属阳，寒邪、湿邪属阴。在疾病的发生发展过程中，邪正相搏导致人体阴阳失调而发生疾病，阴阳失调的基本病机是阴阳偏盛、偏衰和互损等。疾病诊断方面，中医学诊断疾病的过程，包括诊察疾病和辨识证候两个方面。《素问·阴阳应象大论》说："善诊者，察色按脉，先别阴阳。"阴阳学说用于病证诊断，旨在分析四诊所收集的临床资料，从而概括各种病证的阴阳属性。指导疾病防治方面，防治疾病的基本原则是调整阴阳，使脏腑经络、精气血津液、体质恢复相对平衡，达到阴平阳秘的生理状态。

Yin-yang theory has a very special significance and status for traditional Chinese medicine. It runs through the theoretical system of traditional Chinese medicine, which is not only the core concept and basic guiding ideology for the theoretical system construction of traditional Chinese medicine, but also an important theoretical tool for medical practice and theoretical research. *Yin-yang* theory, which is related to traditional Chinese medicine theories such as *zang-xiang*, meridians, pathogenesis, treatment, prescription, acupuncture and health preservation, is also the concrete manifestation of the relationship between traditional Chinese medicine and traditional Chinese culture.

The concept of *yin-yang*, which belongs to the category of ancient Chinese philosophy, is a summary of two opposite aspects of interrelated things. It can represent both the division of properties and movement changes of two related and corresponding things or phenomena, and the properties and movement laws of two opposing aspects within one thing.

The classic expression of the basic concept of *yin* and *yang* in traditional Chinese medicine can be found in the *Yinyang Yingxiang Dalun of Su Wen* (*Major Discussion on the theory of Yin and Yang and the Corresponding Relationships Among All the Things in Nature*, the chapter of *Plain Conversation*): "*Yin* and *yang* serve as the law of the heaven and the earth, the fundamental principle of all things, the parents of change, the beginning of birth and death and the storehouse of *Shenming* (spirit)."

Yin and *yang* are the laws of nature and foundation of the change of all things in the world. They run through the life and death of things, and are the internal driving force for the occurrence, development and change of things.

1 Main Contents of *Yin-Yang* Theory

Yin-yang theory explains the fundamental laws of creation, development and change of things in the universe based on the unity of opposites and interaction of *yin* and *yang*. Its main contents include mutual interaction of *yin* and *yang*, opposition of *yin* and *yang*, interdependence of *yin* and *yang*, waxing and waning between *yin* and *yang*, transformation between *yin* and *yang*, and spontaneous harmonization between *yin* and *yang*, etc.

1.1 Mutual Interaction of *Yin-Yang*

Mutual interaction of *yin-yang* means that *yin* and *yang* mutually affect and interact with one another in the movement. It's the root and basis of the generation and change of things in the universe.

Yang qi raises and accumulates to form the heaven and *yin qi* descends and accumulates to constitute the earth. The heaven *qi* descends and the earth *qi* ascends. They mutually interact with one another, producing all things in the universe. In nature, the mutual interaction of these two kind of *qi* forms clouds, fog, lightning, rain and dew, and all things can be generated.

As one of the species in the universe, human beings are also generated by it. Living things are generated under the interaction of the heaven and the earth, *yin* and *yang*. Without the movement of *yin* and *yang*, there would be no life in the universe.

Mutual interaction of *yin – yang* is the driving force for the development and change of things and phenomena. *Yin* and *yang* have opposite properties, the two continue to mingle with each other and interact with each other. Only in this way can all things in the universe live and change endlessly.

1.2　Opposition of *Yin* and *Yang*

Opposition of *yin* and *yang* means that *yin* and *yang* are the two opposite aspects of things, which is the inherent property of things or phenomena.

Yin – yang theory holds that all things and phenomena in the universe have a dual aspect.

For example, heaven and earth, day and night, water and fire, man and woman, cold and heat, motion and quiet, up and down, left and right, etc.

The form of opposition between *yin* and *yang* plays a role through mutual struggle and mutual restriction between *yin* and *yang*.

Yin can restrain *yang*, while *yang* also can restrain *yin*.

The mutual restriction of *yin* and *yang* is the root of the reciprocal changes of the four seasons.

The normal physiological activities of human body have two states of excitement and inhibition, that is, excitement is *yang* and inhibition belongs to *yin*, which restrict each other.

Yang restricts *yin* in the day, and people are in a state of excitement and soberness.

While at night, *yin* restricts *yang* and people enters a state of sleep.

The opposition between *yin* and *yang* brings about different changes in sleeping and awaking during day and night. The movement and stillness maintain the normal rhythm of people's sleeping and awaking, fully reflecting the mutual opposition and mutual constraints of *yin* and *yang*.

The significance of the opposition between *yin* and *yang* is to prevent either side of *yin* and *yang* from being excess and maintain the coordination and balance between *yin* and *yang*.

The two are always in a contradictory movement. Within a certain limit, they struggle with each other and restrain each other so that neither side is excess nor deficient, so that things or phenomena can remain a dynamic equilibrium within and between each other and thus things can live and develop.

If one of the *yin* and *yang* is excess, the other side is over restricted by it, or if one is too deficient to restrict the other, the opposition and restriction between *yin* and *yang* will be out of balance and the dynamic equilibrium between them will be disrupted. Then diseases arise.

1.3　Interdependence of *Yin* and *Yang*

Interdependence of *yin* and *yang* means that the two opposite aspects of *yin* and *yang*, which are complementary and interdependent.

It works through the form of mutual storing of *yin* and *yang* and mutual rooting of *yin* and *yang*.

1.3.1　Mutual Storing of *Yin* and *Yang*

Mutual storing of *yin* and *yang* means that either of the opposing sides of *yin* and *yang* contains the other side. That is, there is *yin* within *yang* and *yang* within *yin*.

Everything in the universe contains components with different attributes of *yin* and *yang*. Things belonging to *yang* contain *yin* components, while things belonging to *yin* also contain *yang* components.

In terms of the heaven and the earth, the former is *yang* and the latter is yin.

The heaven is formed by the rising *qi* of the earth, so *yin* is contained in *yang*.

And the earth is formed by the descending *qi* of the heaven, so *yang* is contained in *yin*.

1.3.2　Mutual Rooting of *Yin* and *Yang*

Mutual rooting of *yin* and *yang* refers to the fundamental and interdependent relationship between *yin* and *yang*, that is, "the root of *yang* is in *yin*, and the root of *yin* is in *yang*".

Both sides are prerequisites for each other.

The two sides of *yin* and *yang*, which are fundamental to each other, have the role of mutual livelihood, promotion and reinforcement.

The meaning of mutual storing and mutual rooting of *yin* and *yang* lies in the fact that *yin* and *yang* are always unified. Each side takes the existence of the other as a precondition for its own existence, and neither side can exist without the other.

For example, spring and summer are *yang*, autumn and winter are *yin*. Without spring and summer, there would be no autumn and winter, without autumn and winter, there would be no spring and summer.

Cold is *yin*, and heat is *yang*. Without cold, there is no heat, and vice versa.

Yin cannot exist without *yang*, and *yang* cannot exist without *yin*. They are inseparable.

1.4　Waxing and Waning Between *Yin* and *Yang*

Waxing and Waning between *yin* and *yang* means that both *yin* and *yang* are not static, but in the continuous reduction and increase of motion changes.

Waning means reduction and reduction, and waxing means increase and growth.

The ancient philosophers believed that both *yin* and *yang* were in motion all the time. There were dynamic waxing and waning between *yin* and *yang*. The waxing and waning of *yin-yang* maintained a dynamic balance within a certain range, limit, time and space. It was precisely because of the change of *yin* and *yang* that all things in nature can maintain a relative and dynamic balance.

The forms of waxing and waning of *yin-yang* belongs to the movement change in the process of quantitative change, including the mutual waxing and waning of *yin-yang*, and the simultaneous waxing and waning of *yin-yang*.

1.4.1　Mutual Waxing and Waning Between *Yin* and *Yang*

The opposing *yin* and *yang* show mutual waxing and waning in the process of restricting each other. There are two forms of it: one is that one waxes and the other wanes, which refers to the increasing of one side of *yin-yang* and the decreasing of the other side. The other is that one side of *yin-yang* diminishes and the other side increases accordingly. *Yin* and *yang* are mutually restricted, so the dynamic waxing and waning between *yin* and *yang* can occur.

The change of climate and day-night in the four seasons of nature is a reflection of the waxing and waning of *yin* and *yang*.

The physiological activity of the human body is also the embodiment of the waxing and waning of *yin* and *yang*. *yang* is generated at midnight, and *yin* is generated at midday. The physiological functions of the human body also gradually turn excitement to inhibition, that is the process of "*yin* waxing and *yang* waning".

1.4.2　Simultaneous Waxing and Waning Between *Yin* and *Yang*

The interdependent *yin* and *yang* sides have shown changes in the process of mutual promotion.

There are two forms of it: One is that one side of *yin-yang* grows and the other also grows. The other is that one side decreases, and the other side also decreases.

Since *yin* and *yang* interact with each other, *yang* can promote the transformation of *yin* and the waxing of *yin* can promote the generation of *yang*. If *yang* disappears, *yin* cannot be transformed, if *yin* disappears, *yang* cannot generate. The simultaneous waxing and waning of *yin-yang* is a movement change in the interdependence between *yin-yang*, which is realized in the process of waxing and waning of *yin-yang*.

In the climate changes of the four seasons, rainfall gradually increases with the gradual rise of temperature in spring and summer, and decreases with the cooler climate in autumn and winter. That is the manifestation of simultaneous waxing and waning of *yin-yang*.

In human physiological activities, the lack of strength that occurs when you are hungry. That is, due to the lack of essence (*yin*), it cannot generate *qi* (*yang*). This phenomenon is called *yang* disappears with *yin*. While supplement essence (*yin*) to produce energy (*yang*) and increase the strength of human body is called *yang* grows with *yin*.

The meaning of the waxing and waning of *yin-yang* is to maintain the relative and dynamic balance between them.

Within certain limits, the movement of waxing and waning of *yin* and *yang* belong to the normal state.

For example, the cold, heat, warm and cool in nature and the *qi* and blood *yin* and *yang* of the human body are always in the continuous movement and change of *yin* and *yang*, neither deficient nor excess, but maintaining a relative dynamic balance within a certain range.

The movement of *yin* and *yang* in nature is reflected by normal climate changes, while in the human body it is reflected by the normal life activities.

Therefore, the waxing and waning of *yin* and *yang* is absolute, and the balance between *yin* and *yang* is relative. It is extremely important to maintain the dynamic balance between *yin* and *yang* in the process of *yin* and *yang* movement.

1.5　Mutual Transformation of *Yin* and *Yang*

Mutual transformation of *yin-yang* refers to the *yin* and *yang* attributes of things. *Yin* and *yang* can be transformed to the opposite under certain conditions, that is, the things that belong to *yang* can be transformed into the things belong to *yin* and the things that belong to *yin* can be transformed into the things belong to *yang*. The mutual transformation of *yin* and *yang* generally arises from the "extreme" stage of the development and change of things, that is, "Things will develop in the opposite direction when they become extreme." When the movement of *yin* and *yang* develops to a certain stage, changes will occur. When the ratio of *yin* to *yang* within a thing is reversed, the properties of the thing are transformed.

Both the waxing and waning of *yin* and *yang* and mutual transformation of *yin* and *yang* are the manifestations of *yin* and *yang* movement, but the essence is different. The former is a process of quantitative change, and the attributes of things themselves have not changed. The latter is qualitative change based on quantitative change, and the attributes of things themselves are transformed into the opposite side.

The transformation of *yin* and *yang* is the result of the waxing and waning of *yin* and *yang*. The waxing and waning of *yin* and *yang* develops to the extreme period is the condition of transformation. When the movement of *yin* and *yang* exceeds a certain limit, the attribute of the thing will be transformed.

1.6 Spontaneous Harmonization Between *Yin* and *Yang*

Spontaneous harmonization between *yin* and *yang* refers to the ability and tendency for *yin* and *yang* to automatically maintain and restore their coordinated and stable state.

It's the nature of *yin* and *yang*.

Taking "spontaneous" as it's core, it realizes "harmonization" by the interaction of *yin* and *yang*.

The mechanism of spontaneous harmonization between *yin* and *yang* lies in the interaction between them.

Although the attributes of *yin* and *yang* are opposite, there are mutual relationships between the two, such as mutual rooting, mutual transformation, mutual restraint and mutual interaction, which are opposite in the changes of interaction. They are the internal mechanisms for maintaining the coordinated development of things or phenomena.

Yin and *yang* are in relative and dynamic balance. Both *yin* and *yang* are in a state of general equilibrium in their interaction, that is, *yin* and *yang* are in a state of harmony and relative stability. On the basis of mutual rooting and mutual interaction, *yin* and *yang* are opposed and constrained.

They move and change within certain limits and conditions to maintain a balanced state.

2 Current Researches of the Application and Development of *Yin-Yang* Theory

Traditional Chinese medicine uses the *yin-yang* theory to guide the understanding of specific things with dialectical thinking, clarify the physical structure, functional activities, pathological changes, clinical diagnosis, disease prevention and treatment, and health preservation and rehabilitation of life, which lays the foundation of the theoretical system of traditional Chinese medicine.

In terms of explaining the changes of human diseases, the occurrence of diseases marks an imbalance in the coordination between *yin* and *yang*, which is called "disharmony between *yin* and *yang*".

According to the nature and pathogenic characteristics of pathogenic factors, traditional Chinese medicine divides the pathogenic factors into two categories: *yin* and *yang*. For example, it is said in the *Tiaojing Lun of Su Wen* (*Discussion on the Regulation of Channel*, the chapter of *Plain Conversation*) : "The attack of evil may cause diseases of *yang* or diseases of *yin*. "

Generally speaking, the six excesses belong to *yang* evil, emotional disorders, improper diet, irregular living habit belong to *yin* evil.

Among the *yin* evil and *yang* evil, there also have *yin* and *yang*. For example, in the six excesses, wind, summer-heat and fire belong to *yang*, while cold and dampness belong to *yin*.

In the course of the occurrence and progress of the disease, struggle between anti-pathogenic *qi* and pathogenic factors leads to the imbalance of *yin* and *yang* in the human body and causes the disease. The basic pathogenesis of disharmony between *yin* and *yang* are excess *yin* or *yang*, waning of *yin* or *yang* and mutual impairment between *yin* and *yang*.

In terms of disease diagnosis, the process of disease diagnosis in traditional Chinese medicine includes two aspects: diagnosis and pattern differentiation.

It is said in the *Yinyang Yingxiang Dalun of Su Wen* (*Major Discussion on the theory of Yin and Yang and the Corresponding Relationships Among All the Things in Nature*, the chapter of *Plain Conversation*): "The skilled diagnosticians exam the countenance and feel the pulse. They differentiate *yin* and *yang* first."

Yin-Yang theory is used in the diagnosis of patterns, aims to analyze the clinical data collected by the four diagnostic methods so as to summarize the *yin* and *yang* attributes of various diseases.

In the aspect of guiding the prevention and treatment of diseases, the basic principle is to adjust *yin* and *yang*, so that *zang-fu* organs, meridians, essence, *qi*, blood, fluid, and physique can restore relative balance, and achieve the balance of *yin* and *yang*.

第五节 五行学说
(Five-Element Theory)

五行学说是我国古代哲学思想中影响最为广泛的重要学说之一,在中国传统文化中占有重要的历史地位。该学说在被引入中医学指导临床实践的过程中又得到了进一步丰富,不仅成为中医基础理论的核心之一,而且也成为中医学基本思维模式之一。

五行,即木、火、土、金、水五类物质属性及其运动变化。"五",指由宇宙本原之气分化的构成宇宙万物的木、火、土、金、水五类物质属性;"行",指运动变化。从古代哲学概念出发,五行已超越木、火、土、金、水的具体物质,衍化为归纳宇宙万物并阐释其相互关系的五类物质属性。

五行学说是以木、火、土、金、水五类物质属性及其运动规律来认识世界、解释世界和探求宇宙变化规律的世界观和方法论。秦汉之际,五行学说进入广泛应用和发展阶段,用于天文、地理、历法、气象、社会、经济、兵法等各领域,尤以中医学最为突出。古人运用五行学说,采用取象比类和推演络绎的方法,将自然与社会的各种事物或现象分为五类,并以五行之间生克制化关系来解释其发生、发展和变化的规律。

一、五行学说基本内容(Basic Contents of Five-Elements Theory)

五行学说的基本内容包括两个方面:一是五行生克制化的正常规律;二是五行生克的异动变化。

(一)五行生克制化

五行生克制化,是在正常状态下五行系统所具有的自我调节机制。由于五行之间存在着相生、相克与制化的关系,从而维持五行系统的平衡与稳定,促进事物的生生不息。

五行相生,指木、火、土、金、水之间存在着有序的递相资生、助长和促进的关系。五行相生次序是:木生火,火生土,土生金,金生水,水生木。在五行相生关系中,任何一行都具有"生我"和"我生"两方面的关系。《难经》将此关系比喻为母子关系:"生我"者为母,"我生"者为子。因此,五行相生,实际上是五行中的某一行对其子行的资生、促进和助长。以火为例,木生火,故"生我"者为木,木为火之母;火生土,故"我生"者为土,土为火之子。木与火是母子关系,火与土也是母子关系。

五行相克,指木、火、土、金、水之间存在着有序的间相克制、制约和抑制的关系。五行相克次序是:木克土、土克水、水克火、火克金、金克木。在五行相克关系中,任何一行都具有"克我"和"我克"两方面的关系。《黄帝内经》把相克关系称为"所胜""所不胜"关系:"克我"者为我"所不胜","我克"者为我"所胜"。因此,五行相克,实际上是五行中的某一行对其所胜一行的克制和制约。如以木为例,由于木克土,故"我克"者为土,土为木之"所胜";由于金克木,故"克我"者为金,金为木之"所不胜"。

五行制化,制,克制;化,生化。五行制化,指五行之间递相生化,又间相制约,生化中有制约,制约中有生化,二者相辅相成,从而维持其相对平衡和正常的协调关系。五行制化属五行相生与相克相结合的自我调节,是五行系统处于正常状态下的调控机制。五行相生和相克是不可分割的两个方面:没有生,就没有事物的发生和成长;没有克,就不能维持事物间的正常协调关系。因此,必须生中有克,克中有生,相反相成,才能维持事物间的平衡协调,促进稳定有序的变化与发展。

(二)五行生克异常

五行生克关系出现异常包括五行母子相及与相乘相侮。五行之间异常的生克变化,主要用于阐释某些异常的气候变化和人体的病机变化。

1.五行母子相及 五行母子相及属于相生关系的异常变化,包括母病及子和子病及母两种情况。

母病及子,指五行中的某一行异常,累及其子行,导致母子两行皆异常。如肾病及肝,即属母病及子。

子病及母,指五行中的某一行异常,累及其母行,终致子母两行皆异常。子病及母,既有子行不足引起母行亦虚的母子俱虚,又有子行亢盛导致母行亦盛的母子俱实,以及子行亢盛损伤母行,导致子盛母衰,即所谓"子盗母气"。如肝病及肾,即属于病及母。

2.五行相乘相侮　五行相乘相侮,属于相克关系的异常变化,包括相乘和相侮2种情况。

(1)相乘:指五行中某一行对其所胜一行的过度制约或克制。五行相乘的次序与相克相同,即木乘土,土乘水,水乘火,火乘金,金乘木。导致五行相乘的原因有"太过"和"不及"两种情况。太过导致的相乘:五行中的某一行过于亢盛,对其所胜一行进行超过正常限度的克制,引起其所胜一行的虚弱,从而导致五行之间的协调关系失常。不及所致的相乘:五行中某一行过于虚弱,难以抵御其所不胜一行正常限度的克制,使其本身更显虚弱。

相乘与相克虽然在次序上相同,但本质上是有区别的。相克是正常情况下五行之间的制约关系,相乘则是五行之间的异常制约现象。在人体,相克表示生理现象,相乘表示病机变化。

(2)相侮:指五行中某一行对其所不胜一行的反向制约和克制。五行相侮的次序与相克的次序相反,即木侮金、金侮火、火侮水、水侮土、土侮木。

导致五行相侮的原因,亦有"太过"和"不及"两种情况。太过所致的相侮:五行中的某行过于强盛,使原来克制它的一行不仅不能克制它,反而受到它的反向克制。不及所致的相侮:五行中某一行过于虚弱,不仅不能制约其所胜,反而受到其反向克制。

五行相乘和相侮,都是相克关系的异常,两者之间既有区别又有联系。相乘与相侮的主要区别是:前者是按五行的相克次序发生过度的克制,后者是与五行相克次序发生相反方向的克制现象。相乘与相侮的联系是:在发生相乘时,也可同时发生相侮;发生相侮时,也可同时发生相乘。

二、五行学说应用(Application of Five-Elements Theory)

五行学说在中医学的运用,主要是以五行特性来分析和归纳人体的形体结构及生理功能,构建以五脏为中心、与自然环境紧密联系的五脏系统,以说明五脏之间的生理联系,指导疾病的诊断和防治。

五行学说作为中医学主要的认识论,以五行特性类比五脏的生理特点,确定五脏的五行属性,在五脏配属五行基础上,推演络绎人体的各种组织结构与功能,将形体、官窍、情志等分归于五脏,构建以五脏为中心的生理系统。同时,又将自然界的五方、五气、五化、五色、五味等与五脏联系起来,将人体内外环境联结成一个密切联系的整体,形成五脏一体、天人一体的五脏系统,奠定了中医藏象学说的理论基础。中医学根据五行特性,取象比类,将五脏分别归属于五行。如肝气喜条达而恶抑郁,具有面通气血、调畅情志的功能,相应于木之生长、升发、条达的特性,故肝属木;心具有主血脉而动血液运行、主神明为脏腑之大主的功能,相应于火之温热、光明的特性,故心属火;脾具有运水谷、化生精微、为气血生化之源以营养脏腑形体的功能,相应于土之生化万物的特性,故脾属土;肺气肃降,具有主呼吸、通调水道输布水液的功能,相应于金之清肃、收敛的特性,故肺属金;肾具有藏精、主水的功能,相应于水之滋润、下行、闭藏的特性,故肾属水。同时,中医学运用五行生克制化理论,分析五脏之间的主要关系,从而把五脏联系成一个有机的整体,维持人体内环境的统一。

The five-element theory is one of the most widely influential theories in ancient Chinese philosophy, and occupies an important historical position in Chinese traditional culture.

In particular, the theory has been further enriched in the process of clinical practice of traditional Chinese medicine. It has not only become one of the cores of the basic theory of traditional Chinese medicine, but also affected the thinking mode of traditional Chinese medicine.

The five-elements refer to wood, fire, earth, metal and water as well as their motion and changes.

"Five" refers to the five physical attributes of wood, fire, earth, metal and water, which are formed by the original *qi* of the universe.

"*Xing*" refers to the movement and change.

Proceeding from the concept of ancient philosophy, the five-elements have gone beyond the concrete matter of wood, fire, earth, metal and water, and have evolved into five types of material attributes that summarize all things and their interrelations.

The five-element theory is a world outlook and methodology to understand the world, explain the world and explore the laws of cosmic changes based on the five material attributes of wood, fire, earth, metal and water and their laws of movement.

During the Qin and Han dynasties, five-elements theory entered a stage of wide application and development, which was used in astronomy, geography, calendar, meteorology, society, economy, art of war and other fields, especially in traditional Chinese medicine.

The ancient people used this theory, adopted the method of image analogy and deduction, divided various things or phenomena between nature and society into five categories and explained the laws of their occurrence, development and change with the relationship between generation and restriction of the five-elements.

1 Basic Contents of Five-Element Theory

The basic contents of five-element theory includes two aspects: one is the normal law of the generation and restriction of the five-elements, and the other is the abnormal changes of the five-elements.

1.1 Mutual Generation, Controlling, Restriction and Transformation of Five-Elements

The movement of mutual generation, controlling, restriction and transformation of the five-elements is the self-regulation mechanism of the five-elements system in the normal state.

Due to the relationship among the five-elements, the balance and stability of the five-elements system are maintained and things are promoted continuously.

The five-elements mutually generate, which means that there is an orderly relationship between wood, fire, earth, metal and water. They promote the growth of each other.

The generation activity among the five-elements follows a circular order: wood generates fire, fire generates earth, earth generates metal, metal generates water, and water, in turn, generates wood.

In this circular order, each of the five-elements is marked by such relations as "being generated" and "generating".

Nanjing (*Classic of Questioning*) compares this relationship to the relationship between mother and child: Each element is the mother it generates and the child of the element that generates it.

Therefore, generation means that one kind of object generates, strengthens or brings forth the child of it.

Take fire for example, since wood generates fire, it is the mother of fire.

Fire generates earth, so earth is the child of fire.

Wood and fire are mother-child relationship, so as the fire and earth.

Mutual restriction among the five-elements refers to the orderly relationship of mutual restriction and inhibition among wood, fire, earth, metal and water.

The restricting activity among the five-elements follows a circular order: Wood restricts earth, earth restricts water, water restricts fire, fire restricts metal, and metal, in turn, restricts wood. In this circular order, each of the five-elements is marked by "being restricted" and "restricting".

Neijing (*Yellow Emperor's Canon of Medicine*) regards mutual restriction among the five-elements as "being restricted" and "restricting". Therefore, mutual restraint among the five-elements is actually the restraint and restriction of one element on the restricted one.

Take wood for example, since wood restricts earth, the element that is restricted by wood is earth, the restricting element is wood. The element restricting wood is metal, the restricted element is wood.

The five-elements mutually control and transform. It refers to the balanced, harmonized state maintained by mutual generating and restraining relationships among the five-elements. Mutual control and transformation of five-elements is the self-regulation of generation and restriction, and the regulatory mechanism of the five-element system in its normal state.

Mutual generation and restriction of the five-elements are inseparable from each other: Without generation, there will be no occurrence and growth of things; without restriction, the normal coordination between things cannot be maintained. Therefore, in order to maintain a state of balance and harmony and promote stable and orderly change and development of things, generation and restriction must be kept in balance.

1.2   Abnormal State of Mutual Generation and Restriction of Five-Elements

The abnormal changes of mutual generation and restriction of five-elements include the interaction of mother and child diseases, over-restriction and counter-restriction. They are mainly used to explain some abnormal climate changes and pathological changes of human body.

1.2.1   Interaction of Mother and Child Illnesses Among Five-Elements

The interaction of mother and child illnesses belong to the abnormal changes of mutual generation, including two situations: mother passing illness to child and child's illness affecting the mother.

Mother passing illness to child means that the illness in the mother organ is passed to the child organ, leading to the abnormality of both the mother and the child organ. Kidney illness passes to liver is an example.

Child's illness affecting the mother means that the illness in a child organ affects the mother organ, leading to the abnormality of both the mother and the child organ. It includes three aspects, deficiency of both the mother and the child organ due to the deficiency of the child organ, excess of both the mother and the child organ due to the excess of the child organ, and excess of child organ and deficiency of mother organ, which is the so called "child stealing the mother's qi". Liver illness passes to kidney is an example of child's illness affecting the mother.

1.2.2   Over-restriction and Counter-restriction Among Five-Elements

Over-restriction and counter-restriction among five-elements belong to the abnormal changes of mutual restriction, including two situations: over-restriction and counter-restriction.

(1) Over-restriction is the excessive restraint of an element over the element it controls. The order of it is the same as that of restriction. That is, wood over restricts earth, earth over restricts water, water over restricts fire, fire over restricts metal, and metal, in turn, over restricts wood. There are two reasons for it: "excess" and "deficiency". Over-restriction caused by ex-

cess：the element in excess may over-restrict the restricted element and brings on insufficiency of it,leading to disharmony among five-elements. Over-restriction caused by deficiency：The element is too weak to resist the restraint of the counterpart,making itself even weaker.

Although the order of over-restriction is the same as that of restriction,they are different in nature.

Restriction implies bringing under control or restraint in normal circumstances,while over-restriction is the abnormal restriction phenomenon among five-elements.

In human body,restriction represents a physiological phenomenon,and over-restriction indicates pathological changes.

（2）Counter-restriction means that to a restraining element becomes controlled by the element it controls. The direction of counter-restriction is just the opposite to that of restriction. That is,wood counter restricts metal,metal counter restricts fire,fire counter restricts water,water counter restricts earth and earth,in turn,counter restricts wood.

There are also two reasons for the counter-restriction among five-elements："excess" and "deficiency". Counter-restriction caused by excess：It's a condition in which one element is so strong that the restricting element in the regular order fails to restrict it,but is restricted by it. Counter-restriction caused by deficiency：It's a condition in which one element is so weak that it fails to restrict the other in the regular order,but is restricted by the other in the reverse order.

Over – restriction and counter – restriction are anomalous manifestations of the restriction,and there are both differences and relations between them. The main difference between them is that the former is excessive restraint of an element over the element it controls,and the direction of the latter is just opposite to that ofrestriction. The relationship between them is that the two phenomena can occur together.

2　Application of Five-Element Theory

The role of five-elements theory in tradition Chinese medicine is to analyze and summarize the physical structure and physiological functions of the human body in terms of the characteristics of the five-elements,and to build a system of five *zang*-organs centered on the five organs and closely related to the natural environment. This system is used to explain the physiological connection among the five *zang*-organs and guide the diagnosis and prevention of diseases.

As the main epistemology of traditional Chinese medicine,five-elements theory analogizes the physiological characteristics of the five *zang*-organs with the characteristics of the five-elements,determines the attributes of the five organs. On the basis of the five organs belonging to the five-elements, we deduce the structure and functions of the human body and assign the body, organs and emotions to the five organs to build a physiological system centered on them.

At the same time, it connects the five directions, five *qi*, five transformations, five colors and five flavors of nature with the five *zang* organs, linking the internal and external environment of the human body into a whole, forming the viscera system based on harmony of the five *zang*-organs and unity of human and nature. It has laid the theoretical foundation of the theory of visceral manifestation in traditional Chinese medicine.

According to the characteristics of the five-elements, the five viscera are classified as the five-elements in traditional Chinese medicine.

For example, the liver likes free will and hates to be suppressed. It has the functions of ventilating *qi* and blood and regulating the emotions, corresponding to the growth, ascending and striping characteristics of wood, so the liver pertains to wood.

The heart governs the blood, vessels, and the bright spirit, which corresponds to the warm and bright characteristics of fire, so the heart pertains to fire.

The spleen governs transportation and transformation, it transports and transforms the nutrients of the foodstuff, and is the source of *qi* and blood, corresponding to the characteristics of earth, so the spleen pertains to earth.

The lung dominates purification and descent, it controls respiration and regulates waterways, which corresponds to the characteristics of purging and convergence of mental, so the lung pertains to metal.

The kidney stores essence and governs water and fluids. It corresponds to the characteristics of moistening, descending and storing of water, so the kidney pertains to water.

At the same time, traditional Chinese medicine uses the theory of five-elements to analyze the main relations among the five *zang*-organs. It connects the five *zang*-organs into an organic whole and maintain the unity of human internal environment.

第六节　藏象学说
(Visceral Manifestation Theory)

中医基础学科体系包含藏象、诊法、病机、治则、方剂、药物六大范畴,是中医学之魂。藏象学说是基础的基础,代表着中医的本质特点。先哲运用了哲学的阴阳五行方法,观察了与生命相关的 30 多项要素,综合了要素与要素之间错综复杂的相互关系,演绎为不同于西医基础学科体系的中医藏象学说。它的核心不是解剖及其功能,而是与生命相关的要素及其联系。它完整、真实地体现了中医整体系统观、动态平衡观,是人类科学发现、医学进步中无与伦比的独创领域,几千年来成功地指导着中医临床的防病治病。

藏象,又称"脏象",指脏腑生理功能、疾病变化表现于外的征象。"藏象"是中医学特有的概念,与脏器的概念不同。在藏象学说的构建过程中,大体解剖与整体观察以及"以象测藏"等特殊的认识方法,决定了"藏"的概念是在形态结构基础上又赋予了功能系统所形成的认识。

一、藏象学说基本内容(Basic Contents of Visceral Manifestation Theory)

（一）五脏

五脏,即心、肺、脾、肝、肾的合称。五脏的共同生理特点是化生和贮藏精气,并能藏神而称为"神脏",又与时间、空间等环境因素密切相关。五脏虽各有所司,但彼此协调,共同维持生命活动。

心位于胸中,两肺之间,膈膜之上,外有心包络卫护。形态尖圆,如未开之莲蕊。心在五行属火,为阳中之太阳。心系统包括:心藏神,在志为喜,在体合脉,其华在面,在窍为舌,在液为汗,与夏气相通应。心与小肠通过经络构成表里关系。

肺位于胸腔,左右各一,覆盖于心之上。肺有分叶,"虚如蜂巢"。肺经肺系(指气管、支气管等)与喉、鼻相连,故称喉为肺之门户,鼻为肺之外窍。肺在五行属金,为阳中之少阴。肺系统包括肺藏魄,在志为悲(忧),在体合皮,其华在毛,在窍为鼻,在液为涕,与自然界秋气相通应。肺与大肠构成表里关系。肺具有治理调节全身气、血、津液的作用,概括为"肺主治节"。

脾位于腹腔上部,横膈下方,与胃相邻。脾在五行属土,为阴中之至阴。脾系统包括:脾藏意,在志为思,在形体为四肢及肌肉,其华在唇,在窍为口,在液为涎,与长夏之气相通应。脾与胃通过经络构成表里关系。人出生后,生命过程的维持及其所需精气血津液等营养物质的生成,均依赖于脾(胃)运化所化生的水谷精微,故称脾(胃)为"后天之本""气血生化之源"。

肝位于腹腔,横膈之下,右胁之内。肝在五行属木,为阴中之少阳。肝系统包括:肝藏魂,在志为怒,在体合筋,其华在爪,在窍为目,在液为泪,与春气相通应。肝与胆通过经络构成表里关系。肝主疏泄而藏血,调和气血,刚柔相济,肝的疏泄和藏血功能正常,气血充盈,能耐受疲劳,故称肝为"罢极之本"。

肾左右各一,位于腰部脊柱两侧。肾在五行属水,为阴中之太阴。肾系统包括:肾藏志,在志为恐,在体合骨,其华在发,在窍为耳和二阴,在液为唾,与冬气相通应。肾与膀胱通过经络构成表里关系。肾为先天之本,先天指人诞生前的胚胎时期。先天之精,又称"元精",禀受于父母,藏之于肾,为构成胚胎的基本物质和生命来源。临床与遗传有关的先天疾病,皆责之于肾。

(二)六腑

六腑,是胆、胃、小肠、大肠、膀胱、三焦的合称。六腑的生理功能是"传化物",即受盛传化水谷。六腑的生理特点是"泻而不藏""实而不能满"。饮食物入口,通过食管入胃,经胃腐熟,下传于小肠,经小肠的分清泌浊,其清者(精微、津液)由脾吸收,转输布散于全身,供脏腑经络生命活动之需要;其浊者(糟粕)下达于大肠,经大肠的传导,形成粪便排出体外;废液则经肾之气化而形成尿液,通过膀胱,排出体外。饮食物的消化吸收和排泄,须通过消化道的七道门户,称为"七冲门"。

六腑具有通降下行的特性,即每一腑都必须适时排空其内容物,以保持六腑通畅,功能协调,故有"六腑以通为用,以降为顺"之说。

(三)奇恒之府

奇恒之腑,是脑、髓、骨、脉、胆、女子胞的总称。奇恒之腑形态似腑,多为中空的管腔囊状器官;功能似脏,主藏精气而不泻。因其似脏非脏、似腑非腑,异于常态,故以"奇恒"名之。除胆为六腑之外,其余皆无表里配合,也无五行配属,但与奇经八脉有关。

(四)脏腑之间的关系

藏象学说以五脏为中心,以精、气、血、津液为物质基础,通过经络系统,将脏、腑、奇恒之腑沟通联系成有机整体。脏腑之间的关系主要有:脏与脏之间的关系,腑与腑之间的关系,脏与腑之间的关系,脏与奇恒之腑之间的关系。

二、藏象学说应用(Application of Visceral Manifestation Theory)

中医学诊断疾病的过程包括中医的诊法与辨证2个步骤。而藏象理论在其中起着重要的指导作用。

(一)藏象理论与诊法

中医学以五脏为中心,将人体所有的器官、组织建立起各有所属的相互联系,使机体形成内外统一的整体。当内在脏腑发生病变,必然会有相应的症状和体征表现出来,所谓"有诸内必形诸外"。中医诊断疾病主要包括望、闻、问、切四种方法。通过对患者做全面的诊查,并且对相应病史的询问,从其表现出来的各种症状和体征等方面,推测内在脏腑的病理变化,从而对病因、病位和病性做出正确判断。

(二)藏象学说与辨证

中医的辨证主要是通过分析四诊资料,对疾病的病位、病性、病势以及转归趋势进行判断的一个过程。虽然辨证分为八纲辨证、脏腑辨证、卫气营血辨证、三焦辨证等多种方法,但最终还是要以脏腑经络辨证为基础。脏腑是构成人体的一个有密切联系的整体,五脏之间有生克乘侮的关系,脏腑之间有互为表里的联系,疾病演变过程中虚实寒热参合更迭,反映出来的病理变化和证候极为错综复杂。然而只要掌握了脏腑生理病理的内涵和特点,结合四诊八纲进行辨证,可执简驭繁,有助于对病位、病性和转归预后等进行了解。

（三）藏象学说与中医治疗

藏象理论是创立各种治疗方法的理论基础,脏腑生理功能和病理变化是确立治法的理论依据。中医学在确立治疗方法时要以脏腑的生理功能及特性作为基础。如胃为阳腑,具有"传化物而不藏"的功能,其特性是"以通为用,以降为顺"。因此临床上常常会出现"胃气上逆"的症状,如脘痞、呃逆、呕吐、嗳气等。此时治疗的原则就要顺应胃腑的特性,采用通降的方法。

在临床处方时,既要针对主要病机,也要充分考虑到脏腑的生理功能和特性,这样才能收到较好的疗效。

The basic science system of traditional Chinese medicine includes six categories: visceral manifestation, diagnostic methods, pathogenesis, treatment principles, prescription, and medicine. It is the soul of traditional Chinese medicine.

It's the foundation of traditional Chinese medicine and represents the essential characteristics of traditional Chinese medicine.

The ancient philosophers used the philosophical method of *yin-yang* and five-elements to observe more than 30 elements related to life, synthesized the intricate relationship between them, finally formed the visceral manifestation theory in traditional Chinese medicine, which is different from the basic scientific system of western medicine.

Its core is not anatomy and its function, but the elements related to life and their relations.

This theory completely and truly embodies the concept of correspondence between man and nature, the view of whole system and the view of dynamic balance in traditional Chinese medicine. It is an unparalleled and original field of human scientific development and medical progress, and has successfully guided the clinical prevention and treatment of diseases in TCM for thousands of years.

Visceral manifestation, also known as "*zang-xiang*", refers to exterior manifestations of physiological function and pathological changes of internal organs. It's a unique concept of traditional Chinese medicine, which is different from that of organs. In the process of constructing visceral manifestation theory, the special cognitive methods such as anatomy and overall observation as well as "differentiate *zang*-organs (internal organs) by *xiang* (manifestation)" determine that the concept of "*zang*" is endowed with the understanding formed by the functional system on the basis of morphological structure.

1 Basic Contents of Visceral Manifestation Theory

1.1 Five *Zang*-Organs

The five *zang*-organs are the heart, lung, spleen, liver and kidney. The common physiological function of the five *zang*-organs is to transform and store essence. The five *zang* organs are called *Shenzang* because they all have the function of storage *Shen* (spirit). They are also closely related to environmental factors such as time and space. Although the five *zang*-organs govern different parts, they coordinate with each other to maintain life activities together. The heart is located in the chest, between the lungs, above the diaphragm, and protected by the pericardium. Just like the unopened lotus stamen. The heart pertains to fire in the five-elements, which is *Taiyang* within *yang*. The heart system: Heart stores spirit and represents joy in emotions. The vessels are the tissue of the heart, the lustre shows in the face, and the fluid is sweat. It connects the tongue in orifices and is related to summer-*qi*. The heart is internally and externally related to the small instestine.

The lungs are located in the thoracic cavity, one on the left and one on the right, covering the heart. The lungs have lobes, and hollow like a beehive. The lung is connected to the throat and nose through the lung system (trachea, bronchus, etc.), so the throat is called the portal of the lung, and the nose is the external orifice of the lung. The lung is pertains to metal in the five-elements, which is the *Shaoyin* within *yang*. The lung system: The lung stores the Corporeal Soul and represents grief in emotions. The outer aspect of the lung is the skin, the lustre shows in the body hair, and the fluid is nasal discharge. It connects the nose in orifices and is related to autumn-*qi*. The lung is internally and externally related to the large intestine. The lung has the function of regulating *qi*, blood and body fluids in the body, which can be summarized as the "the lung governs management and regulation".

The spleen is located at the upper part of the abdominal cavity, below the diaphragm, and adjacent to the stomach. The spleen pertains to the earth in the five-elements, which is the most yin within *yin*. The spleen system: Spleen stores thought and represents thinking in emotions. It governs the limbs and muscles. The lustre shows in the lips and the fluid is saliva. It connects mouth in orifices and is related to late summer-*qi*. The spleen is internally and externally related to stomach. The spleen and stomach transport nutrients of the foodstuff to generate essence, *qi*, blood and body fluids needed to sustain life activities, so the spleen and stomach are considered as the postnatal foundation and the source of *qi* and blood.

The liver is located in the abdominal cavity, below the diaphragm and within the right hypochondrium. The liver pertains to wood in the five-elements, and it is the *Shaoyang* witnin *yin.* The liver system:Liver stores ethereal soul and represents anger in emotions. The tissue of the liver is sinew,the lustre shows in the nails and the fluid are tears. It connects eyes in orifices and is related to spring-*qi*. The spleen is internally and externally related to the gallbladder. The liver governs the free flow of *qi* and stores blood. It regulates *qi* and blood. When it functions well and the *qi* and blood are full,people can withstand fatigue. So the liver is the foundation for fatigue endurance.

The kidneys,one on the left and one on the right,lie on both sides of the lumbar spine. Kidney pertains to water in five-elements,which is *Taiyin* within yin. Kidney system:Kidney stores will and represents fear in emotions. The kidney governs the bones. The lustre shows in the hair and the fluid is thick saliva. It opens into the urethra and anus and is related to winter-*qi*. The kidney is internally and externally related to the bladder. Kidney is the congenital foundation. Congenital period refers to the period of embryo before the birth of a person. The innate essence,also known as "Yuan-original essence",is inherited from one's parents and stored in the kidney. It is the basic substance of life,which contributes to the generation of offspring. Clinically,congenital diseases associated with heredity all originate from the kidney.

1.2 Six *Fu*-Organs

The six *fu*-organs,including the gallbladder,stomach,small intestine,large intestine,bladder and *sanjiao*. The physiological function of the six *fu*-organs is to receive,transport and transform water and food. And the physiological characteristics of the six *fu*-organs are "receiving food but not storing essence" and "being solid but not full". Food enters the stomach through the esophagus. It is digested by the stomach,and is passed down to the small intestine. Through the small intestine,the clear (essence and body fluids) is absorbed by the spleen and transferred to the whole body for the needs of the vital activities of the internal organs and meridians. The turbid (dregs) reaches the large intestine,and through the conduction of the large intestine,it forms excrement and is excreted to the body. The waste liquid is transformed by the kidney and forms urine,which is excreted through the bladder. The digestion,absorption and excretion of food must pass through the seven portals of the digestive tract,which is called "*Qichongmen*".

The six *fu*-organs have the characteristic of residue descending. Each *zang-fu* organ must be emptied of its contents in time to keep the six *fu*-organs smooth and function coordinated. Just like it goes "The six *fu*-organs can function well only through descending and unobstruction".

1.3 Extraordinary *Fu*-Organs

The extraordinary *fu*-organs is a collective term for brain,marrow,bone,vessels,gallbladder and uterus.

The shape of the extraordinary *fu*-organs is similar to that of the *fu*-organs, and most of them are hollow tubular saclike organs.

It only stores essence but not excretes.

Because it seems to be *zang*-organs and *fu*-organs but doesn't pertains to them, and different from the normal state, so it is named "*qiheng* (extraordinary)".

Except for gallbladder, there is no internal and external relations with six *fu*-organs, and there is no distribution with the five-elements. But they are related to the eight extra meridians.

1.4 Relationship Among *Zang-Fu* Organs

Theory of visceral manifestation takes the five *zang* – organs as the center and the essence, *qi*, blood and body fluids as the material basis. Through the meridian system, *zang*-organs, *fu*-organs and the extraordinary *fu*-organs are connected into an organic whole.

The relationship among viscera mainly includes: the relationship among *zang*-organs, the relationship among *fu*-organs, the relationship between *zang*-organs and *fu*-organs, and the relationship between *zang*-organs and the extraordinary *fu*-organs.

2 Application of Visceral Manifestation Theory

The process of diagnosis of disease in traditional Chinese medicine includes two steps: Disease diagnosis and pattern differentiation.

The theory of visceral manifestation plays an important guiding role in it.

2.1 Visceral Manifestation Theory and Diagnostic Methods

In traditional Chinese medicine, all organs and tissues of the human body are interconnected with each other to form a unified whole inside and outside the body. When pathological changes occur in the internal organs, there are bound to be corresponding symptoms and signs. This is called "viscera inside the body must manifest themselves externally." The diagnostic methods in traditional Chinese medicine mainly include inspection, listening and smelling, inquiry as well as palpation. Through a comprehensive examination of the patient, the inquiry of corresponding medical history and the various symptoms and signs, doctors can speculate the pathological changes of the internal viscera and make a correct judgment on the etiology, location and nature of the disease.

2.2 Visceral Manifestation Theory and Pattern Differentiation

Pattern differentiation in traditional Chinese medicine is a process of judging the location, nature, potential and trend of disease through analysing the data collected by four diagnostic methods.

Although pattern differentiation includes a variety of methods, such as pattern differentiation of eight principles, pattern differentiation of *zang–fu* organs, pattern differentiation of *wei*–defence, *qi*, *ying* nutrients and blood, as well as pattern diferentiation of three *Jiao*, pattern differentiation of *zang–fu* organs and meridians are the basis of it. The internal organs make the human body a closely connected whole. The five internal organs have the relations of generation, restriction, over–restriction and counter–restriction, and each *zang*–organ is internally and externally related to a certain *fu*–organ. Deficiency, excess, cold and heat are combined and changed in the progress of disease, reflecting extremely complex pathological changes and symptoms. However, by grasping the connotation and characteristics of the physio–pathology of the internal organs and combining the four diagnostic methods and eight principles to differentiate the patterns, doctors can treat diseases directly, which are helpful to understand the location, nature and prognosis of the disease.

2.3　Visceral Manifestation Theory and Treatment in TCM

Visceral manifestation theory is the theoretical basis for creating various therapeutic methods, while physiological function and pathological changes of viscera are the theoretical basis for establishing the law. Therefore, the physiological functions and characteristics of the internal organs should be used as the basis for determining the treatment method. For example, the stomach pertains to *yang*, which has the function of "transporting and transforming food but not storing", its characteristic is that "it can function well only through unobstruction and descending." Therefore, there are often symptoms of "counter flow rise of stomach *qi*" in clinic, such as fullness in the stomach, hiccup, vomiting and ructus, etc. For these symptoms, the principle of treatment should conform to the characteristics of the stomach and adopt the method of unobstructing and descending. In clinical prescription, doctors should not only aim at the main pathogenesis, but also fully consider the physiological functions and characteristics of the viscera, so as to obtain a better curative effect.

第七节　精、气、血、津液、神
（Essence, *Qi*, Blood, Body Fluids and Spirit）

　　精、气、血、津液是构成和维持人体生命活动的基本物质。精、气、血、津液既是脏腑、经络、形体、官窍等功能活动的产物，又是其功能活动的物质基础。神，是人体生命活动的主宰及其外在总体表现的统称。神以精、气、血、津液为物质基础，又对这些基本物质的生成、运行及功能等发挥调节作用。

一、精、气、血、津液、神概念（Concept of Essence, *Qi*, Blood, Body Fluids and Spirit）

（一）精

人体之精有广义、狭义之分，广义之精包括气、血、津液等人体一切精微物质；狭义之精专指生殖之精。

精是构成和维持人体生命活动的最基本物质，是人体生命的本原。精，贮藏于脏腑、形体、官窍之中，并流动于脏腑、形体、官窍之间。中医学关于精的理论，受到古代哲学精气学说的深刻影响，但又与之有着严格的区别：古代哲学精气学说以精或精气为构成宇宙万物的本原；而人体之精是构成和维持人体生命活动的精微物质及生命繁衍的根源。

（二）气

气是人体内活力很强、运动不息的极细微物质，是构成和维持人体生命活动的基本物质。中医学关于气的理论，受到古代哲学气一元论的深刻影响，但其所论主要是人体之气以及与自然界相关联的气，在研究对象和范围上与古代哲学气一元论有着显著的区别。此外，在中医学术语中，气在不同语境下表达不同的意义。如六气指风、寒、暑、湿、燥、火6种正常的气候变化，邪气指各种致病因素的统称，药物之气指药性等。

（三）血

血，即血液，是行于脉中，循环流注于全身，具有营养和滋润作用的红色液态物质。脉是血液运行的管道，故称为"血府"。血必须在脉中正常运行，才能发挥其生理功能。如因某种原因，血液在脉中运行迟缓涩滞，停积不行则成瘀血。若因外伤等原因，血液逸出脉外而出血，则称为"离经之血"。离经之血若不能及时排出或消散，则成为瘀血，既丧失了血液的生理功能，又可导致新的病机变化。

（四）津液

津液，包括津和液，是人体一切正常水液的总称，包括脏腑、形体、官窍的内在液体及其正常的分泌物。

津和液在性状、分布和功能上有所不同：质地较清稀，流动性较大，布散于体表皮肤、肌肉和孔窍，并能渗入血脉，主要起滋润作用的称为津；质地较浓稠，流动性较小，灌注于骨节脏腑、脑、髓等，主要起濡养作用的称为液。津与液虽有一定的区别，但两者同源于饮食水谷，生成于脾胃，并可相互渗透补充，所以津液常并称，不进行严格区分。津与液的区别，主要用于临床对津液损耗而出现"伤津""脱液"病机变化的分辨。

（五）神

人体之神有广义、狭义之分。广义之神,指人体生命活动的主宰及其外在总体表现的统称,包括形色、眼神、言谈、表情、应答、举止、精神、情志、声息、脉象等方面;狭义之神,指意识、思维、情志等精神活动。神依附于形体而存在。形为神之质,神为形之用。形存则神存。形亡则神灭。

二、精、气、血、津液、神基本内容及应用(Basic Contents and Applications of Essence, *Qi*,Blood,Body Fluids and Spirit)

（一）精

1. 人体之精的生成、贮藏和输泄　人体之精由禀受于父母的先天之精及来源于吸入清气与水谷精微的后天之精相融合而生成。人体之精贮藏于脏腑身形中。肾所藏先天之精,作为生命本原,在胎儿时期便贮藏于肾中。后天之精则经由脾、肺等输送到各脏腑,化为各脏腑之精,并将部分输送于肾中,以充养肾所藏的先天之精。精的输泄主要形式:一是分藏于各脏腑,濡养脏腑,并化气以推动和调节其功能活动;二是生殖之精的施泄以繁衍生命。

2. 人体之精的功能　精宜闭藏而静谧,相对于气之运行不息,其性属阴,具有重要的生理功能。如繁衍生命、生长发育、化生气血、濡养、化身、抗邪作用。

（二）气

1. 人体之气的变化与运动　人体之气是运动不息的,生命过程即是气的运动及其所产生的各种变化的过程。气的运动称为气机。人体之气不断运动,流行全身,内至五脏六腑,外达筋骨皮毛,推动人体的各种生理活动。气化,指气的运动所产生的各种变化,在人体具体表现为精、气、血、津液等生命物质的生成及其相互转化过程。

2. 人体之气的功能　气具有非常重要的作用,是人之根本。起到推动、温煦、防御、固摄、中介的作用。

（三）血

1. 血的运行　血液运行于脉中,循环不已,流布全身,其正常运行受多种因素影响,同时也是多个脏腑共同作用的结果。血的运行有赖于气的推动、温煦和固摄作用。气的推动作用,是血液运行的动力。血行脉中,脉为血府,脉道完好无损和通畅无阻,也是保证血液正常运行的重要因素。血的运行还与血液的清浊状态相关。若血液中痰浊较甚或血液稠浊,可致血行不畅而瘀滞。

血液的正常运行,主要与心、肺、肝、脾等脏的功能密切相关。

心气推动、肺气宣降、肝气疏泄是推动血液运行的重要因素,脾统血、肝藏血则是固摄血液运行的重要因素。心、肺、肝、脾等脏生理功能相互协调、密切配合,共同维持血液的正常运行。

2. 血的功能　血液具有濡养和化神两大功能。

（四）津液

1. 津液的生成、输布和排泄　津液的生成、输布和排泄三大环节涉及多个脏腑的生理功能，是多个脏腑相互协调配合的结果。

津液来源于饮食水谷，在脾胃运化及有关脏腑的共同参与下生成。脾输布津液主要有两条途径：一是将津液上输于肺，通过肺气的宣发肃降，使津液输布于全身而灌溉脏腑、形体和官窍。二是直接将津液输布于全身，即"灌溉四傍"。肝调畅气机以行水。肝主疏泄，调畅气机，气行则津布。三焦决渎为水道。三焦水道通利，津液得以正常输布。津液的正常输布是多个脏腑密切协调、相互配合的结果，是人体生理活动的综合体现。津液的排泄主要通过排出尿液和汗液来完成。此外，呼气和粪便也带走部分津液。与津液的排泄相关的脏主要有肾、肺、脾，由于尿液是津液排泄的最主要途径，因此肾的生理功能在津液排泄中最为重要。

2. 津液的功能　津液的生理功能主要有滋润濡养和充养血脉 2 个方面。

（五）神

1. 神的生成　先天之神，称为"元神"，是神志活动的原动力，由先天精气所生，为生命之根本。精、气、血、津液是神产生的物质基础。精、气、血、津液不仅是构成和维持人体生命活动的基本物质，也是神赖以产生的物质基础。五脏内藏精、气、血、津液，故五脏皆藏神。五脏精、气、血、津液充盈，则五神安藏守舍；五脏精、气、血、津液亏虚，不能化生或涵养五神，则神志活动异常。

2. 神的功能　神对人体生命活动具有重要的调节作用，能够主宰生命活动，主宰精神活动，调节精、气、血、津液，调节脏腑功能。

Essence, qi, blood and body fluids are the basic substances that constitute and maintain human life activities.

Essence, qi, blood and body fluids are not only the products of functional activities such as viscera, meridians, body as well as sense organs and orifices, but also the material basis of their functional activities.

Spirit is a general term for the domination of human life activities and outer manifestation reflecting the life activities.

Spirit takes essence, qi, blood and body fluid as the material basis, and plays a regulatory role in the formation, movement and function of these basic substances.

1 Concept of Essence, *Qi*, Blood, Body Fluids and Spirit

1.1 Essence

The essence of the human body has a broad and narrow meaning.

The essence of the broad sense includes all subtle substances of the human body, such as *qi*, blood, body fluids, etc. The essence of narrow sense refers to the essence of reproduction.

Essence is the most basic substance that constitutes and maintains human life activities, and it is the origin of human life. Essence is stored in the viscera, body, sense organs and orifices, and it flows among them. The theory of essence in traditional Chinese medicine is deeply influenced by the theory of essence *qi* in ancient philosophy, but it is also strictly different from it. The theory of essence *qi* in ancient philosophy takes essence or essence *qi* as the origin of all things in the universe. While the essence of the human body is the nutrients that constitute and maintain the activities of the human body and the source of life reproduction.

1.2 *Qi*

Qi is a substance with strong vitality in human body, and it is a basic substance that constitutes and maintains human life activities. The theory of *qi* in traditional Chinese medicine is deeply influenced by the ancient philosophy of *qi*-monism, but its theory is mainly about the *qi* of human body and the *qi* related to nature, which is significantly different from the ancient philosophy of *qi* - monism in terms of research object and scope. In addition, in TCM terminology, *qi* can be interpreted into different meanings in different contexts. For example, six *qi* refers to the six normal climate changes of wind, cold, summer, dampness, dryness and fire. Pathogenic *qi* refers to the general name of various pathogenic factors. And the *qi* of drugs refers to medicinal properties.

1.3 Blood

Blood is a red liquid substance rich in nutrients and moistening, and it circulates in the vessels. Veins are the pipes through which blood flows, so they are called "house of blood". Blood can perform its physiological functions only if it runs properly in the veins. If the blood runs slowly and stagnantly in the vessels, it will become blood stasis. Blood that has escaped from the vessels due to trauma is called "blood circulating out of meridians". If it cannot be discharged or dissipated in time, it will become blood stasis, which not only loses the physiological function of the blood, but also can lead to new pathological changes.

1.4 Body Fluids

Body fluids are a collective term for all kinds of normal liquids in the body, including internal fluids and secretions of various organs and tissues, such as viscera, body, sense organs and orifices.

According to the difference in quality, function and distribution, it is subdivided into two, Jin (thin fluid) and Ye (thick fluid). Generally speaking, thin fluid mainly spreads in the skin, muscles and orifices, and penetrates into the vessels as a component of blood, which mainly plays a role in moistening. Thick fluid supports in the skeleton, joints, viscera and brain, mainly plays a role in nou-rishing. Although there are some differences between Jin (thin fluid) and Ye (thick fluid), both are derived from food that is transported and transformed in spleen and stomach. The two can penetrate and supplement each other, so they are often called together and does not be strictly distinguished. The difference between Jin (thin fluid) and Ye (thick fluid) is mainly used to discriminate the pathological changes of "damage to thin body fluid" and "exhaustion of thick body fluid" caused by the loss of body fluids.

1.5   Spirit

The spirit of the human body has a broad and narrow sense. In a broad sense, spirit refers to the dominance of life activities and the overall outer manifestations, including posture, complexion, eyes, speech, expression, response, behavior, spirit, emotion, sound, pulse, etc. Spirit in a narrow sense refers to consciousness, thinking, emotion and other spiritual acti-vities. Spirit is attached to the body. Body is the essence of spirit, and spirit is the use of body. The two are interdependent and co−existent.

2   Basic Contents and Applications of Essence, Qi, Blood, Body Fluids and Spirit

2.1   Essence

2.1.1   Generation, Storage and Transportation of Essence

The essence of the human body is derived from the innate essence inherited from one's parents and the acquired essence obtained through clear qi and food nutrients. The essence is stored in the viscera and the body. The innate essence stored in the kidney is the origin of life. It is inherited from one's parents. The acquired essence is conveyed to the viscera through the spleen and lungs, and transformed into the essence of each viscera. The acquired essence is conveyed to the viscera through the spleen and lungs, and transformed into the essence of each viscera. Part of the acquired essence is conveyed to the kidney to enrich the innate essence.

There are mainly two forms of essence transmission and discharge. One is to divide and store in each viscera, moisten and nourish the viscera, and transform *qi* to promote and regulate its functional activities. The other is to release the reproductive essence to multiply life.

2.1.2 Function of Essence

Essence governing storage and stay inside.

Compared with the continuous movement of *qi*, it pertains to *yin* and has important physiological functions, such as reproducing life, growing and developing, generating *qi* and blood, nourishing, embodying and resisting pathogenic factors.

2.2 Qi

2.2.1 Changes and Movements of *Qi*

Qi is constantly moving in human body, and the process of life is the movement of *qi* and the process of various changes it generates. The movement of *qi* is called *qi* activity. *Qi* in the human body constantly moves and is transformed all over the body, ranging from the internal organs to the external skins to promote various physiological activities of the human body. *Qi* transformation refers to various changes produced by *qi* movement, which are embodied in the production of essence, *qi*, blood, body fluids and other living substances and their mutual transformation processes.

2.2.2 Function of *Qi*

Qi is the foundation of human beings. It plays the role of promotion, warmth, protection, securing, and mediation.

2.3 Blood

2.3.1 Circulation of Blood

Blood runs in the pulse, circulates endlessly, and spreads throughout the body. Its normal circulation is affected by many factors, and it is also the result of the joint action of viscera. The circulation of blood depends on the promotion, warmth and securing of *qi*. The promoting action of *qi* is the driving force of blood movement. Blood circulates in the vessels, the vessels are blood house. The intact and unobstructed vessel is also an important factor in ensuring blood flow. Blood circulation is also associated with the turbidity of the blood. If the blood is turbid, it can cause restricted blood circulation and blood stasis.

The normal circulation of blood is closely related to the functions of heart, lung, liver, spleen and other organs.

Promotion of heart *qi*, descending of lung *qi* and transportation of liver *qi* are important factors to promote blood circulation. Spleen governs blood and liver stores blood are two important factors to promote blood flow. The physiological functions of heart, lung, liver and spleen coordinate and cooperate closely with each other to maintain the normal circulation of blood.

2.3.2　Function of Blood

Blood has two functions of nourishing and transforming spirit.

2.4　Body Fluids

2.4.1　Production, Distribution and Excretion of Body Fluids

The three major aspects of the production, distribution and excretion of body fluids involve the physiological functions of multiple viscera. They are the results of mutual coordination and coordination of the viscera.

The body fluids are derived from the food that is transported and transformed by the spleen and stomach. There are two main ways for spleen to transfer body fluids: one is to transfer body fluids to the lung, and the other purge and descend through the circulation of lung qi. The liver regulates qi movement to promote the transportation of body fluids. The liver is in charge of coursing and draining. It can regulate qi movement so that the body fluids can distribute normally.

Sanjiao are the passways of body fluids. The body fluids can be distributed normally only when the passway is unobstructed. The normal distribution and transportation of body fluids is the result of close coordination and mutual coordination of multiple viscera, which is the comprehensive embodiment of human physiological activities. The excretion of body fluids is accomplished mainly by urine and sweat. In addition, breathing and excreta also take away part of the body fluids. Kidney, lung and spleen are the main organs related to the excretion of body fluids. Because urine is the most important way of fluid excretion, the physiological function of kidney is the most important in fluid excretion.

2.4.2　Function of Body Fluids

The physiological functions of body fluids mainly include moistening, nourishing and enriching the blood and vessels.

2.5　Spirit

2.5.1　Origin of Spirit

The innate spirit, called "*Yuanshen* (original spirit)", is the motive force of the spiritual activities, which is born of innate essence and is the foundation of life.

Essence, qi, blood and body fluids are not only the basic substances that constitute and maintain human life activities, but also the material basis of spirit. The five $zang$-organs contain essence, qi, blood and body fluid, so all the five $zang$-organs can store spirit. When essence, qi, blood and body fluid are full in the five $zang$-organs, the five spirits are in harmony. But when they are deficient and cannot transform or nurture five spirits, the mental activity will be abnormal.

2.5.2　Function of Spirit

Spirit has an important regulating effect on human life activities. It can dominate life activities and spiritual activities, regulate essence, blood and body fluids, as well as viscera functions.

第四章

中医日常保健技术
(Daily Health Care Techniques in Traditional Chinese Medicine)

中医是中华民族的瑰宝,它是一门古老而又神奇的医学,是中国人民在防病治病、养生保健的长期实践中不断积累和总结而形成的具有独特风格的医学科学体系。随着社会的不断发展,人们生活水平和保健意识的不断提升,传统的中医日常保健技术慢慢地被人们所接受,走入了我们的生活。中医保健技术虽然是我们的国宝,但是大多数人却都不曾真正地认识过它。因而学习按摩、艾灸、刮痧、拔罐、中医传统运动等中医保健技术的相关原理、操作要点、注意事项,可以更好地帮助人们了解中医、认识中医。

Traditional Chinese Medicine is a treasure of the Chinese nation. It is an ancient and magical medicine that has been continuously accumulated and summarized by the Chinese people in their long – term practice of disease prevention, treatment, and health preservation to form a unique medical scientific system. With the continuous development of society and the improvement of people's living standards and health awareness, Chinese daily health care technology is gradually being accepted by people and has entered in our lives. Although this healthcare technology is our national treasure, most people have never truly recognized it. This chapter will summarize the Chinese non – medical daily health care techniques with the function of health preservation, such as massage, moxibustion, scraping, cupping, traditional Chinese exercises, etc. Further more, this chapter will introduce the relevant principles, operating points, precautions, and other aspects of healthcare technology to help people understand and learn about traditional Chinese medicine, in order to strengthen people's healthy body.

第一节　推　拿
(*Tuina*)

推拿是指在人体经络腧穴及一定部位上施以特定的操作手法或肢体活动,用以保健、治病的方法,又称按摩、乔摩、矫摩等。可疏通经络,滑利关节,促使气血运行,调整脏腑功能,增强人体抗病能力,达到治病防病的目的,广泛应用于临床各科的多种病症中。

　　"推"和"拿"均是推拿学中最常用、最具代表性的手法;手法和功法是推拿学的重要内容和主要治疗技术。推拿疗法除用于保健养生、减肥美容、消除疲劳外,在临床上还广泛用于脊柱骨盆、骨伤、内、妇、儿和五官等科的许多疾病的治疗中。人们习惯性将用于医疗的手法称为"推拿",用于保健的称为"按摩",中医将二者统称为"推拿"。

　　推拿是人类最古老的一门艺术,起源于远古时期,拥有悠久的历史,是祖国传统医学中的一颗璀璨明珠,推拿最早起源于人们进行的自我防护。远古人类进行艰苦的劳动生产过程中常常会发生跌损和疼痛,当身体出现某种部位的不适时,人们会不自觉地进行抚摩、按压,从而发现疼痛得到了缓解,于是逐渐产生了对推拿的认识。经过千百次的重复,远古人类认识到以合适的按压方式,作用于某些部位,可以减轻或消除病痛,因此逐渐地应用于日常活动和医疗行为中,产生了原始的推拿。秦晋汉时期,推拿疗法已摆脱了经验医学的桎梏,成为一门具有民族特色和理论基础的学科,在中医学中占有重要地位。

一、推拿原理（Principle of *Tuina*）

　　推拿其实就是通过不同的手法作用于人体的肌表,通过经络穴位的作用来达到各个脏腑和相应的组织器官间的平衡,加速机体的新陈代谢,修复各种身体上的损伤,从而达到调整人体生理、病理状态以及治病和保健的作用。推拿的作用原理与各种手法有密切关系,其理论依据是中医经络学说。推拿也可通过外力作用,纠正解剖部位的异常,尤其是关节错位、肌腱滑脱等因解剖部位异常而致的病症。

二、推拿作用（Function of *Tuina*）

　　推拿的作用主要是能够缓解人们的紧张以及疼痛。利用按摩推拿可以让气血正常运行,改善身体血液循环,疏通经络,减轻身体的疼痛。

　　（一）疏通经络,调和气血

　　气为血帅,血为气母,气行则血行,气滞则血瘀,血瘀而气亦滞。推拿手法作用于体表经络上,产生局部反应,起到激发和调整经气的作用,推拿通过调畅气机,活血通脉,对失调的内在进行适当的调整,使血脉通道畅通和气推动固摄功能正常,从而起到积极的治疗作用。《黄帝内经》里说"经络不通,病生于不仁,治之以按摩",说明按摩有疏通经络的作用。从生理学的角度来看,通过按摩体表,对机体产生了一定的刺激。通过刺激末梢神经,促进血液、淋巴循环及组织间的代谢过程,以协调各组织、器官间的功能,使机能的新陈代谢水平有所提高。

　　（二）理筋整复,消肿止痛

　　推拿所治之病,多为跌仆闪挫之症,推拿通过拔伸、屈曲、推、按、扳、摇等手法在病变局部和远隔部位的经络腧穴进行操作,通过外力直接作用使关节归正,经脉顺畅,能使损伤得到修复,错缝或脱位得到复位,变位、滑脱畸形得到矫正,从而发挥理筋整复、消肿止痛的作用,恢复人体正常的生活起居和运动功能。

（三）散寒除痹、滑利关节

《素问·痹论》篇中记载:"风寒湿三气杂至,合而为痹也,其风气胜者为行痹,寒气胜者为痛痹,湿气胜者为著痹也……痹在于骨则重,在于脉则血凝而不流,在于筋则屈不伸,在于肉则不仁,在于皮则寒。"按摩具有舒筋通络、利关节、和血脉而除痹痛的作用。风寒湿邪痹阻经脉,阻碍气血运行,导致肌肉、筋骨和关节酸痛、麻木、重着或关节肿胀、变形、活动障碍,甚至引起脏腑功能异常。推拿通过按摩手法,对粘连而僵硬的关节起到松解粘连、滑利关节的作用,对局部软组织变性者,则可改善局部营养供应,促进新陈代谢,从而使变性的组织逐渐得到改善或恢复。

三、推拿基本手法（Basic Manipulations of *Tuina*）

推拿手法各种各样,并不一致,推拿手法也不是单纯孤立地使用,常常是几种手法相互配合进行的,手法要持久、有力、均匀、柔和。归纳起来,常用手法可选如下 8 种。

（一）打

即叩打,用手指、手掌或拳叩打,分为用掌打、用拳打。打法手劲要轻重有准,柔软而灵活。手法合适,能给患者以轻松感,否则就是不得法。叩打时间一般是 1 ~ 2 分钟,或 3 分钟就可以了。极个别情况下,根据病情,延长一些时间或缩短一些时间。这种手法也可在按摩后来配合进行,也可同其他按摩手法夹杂进行。

（二）颤

即颤动,用手指端或手掌轻微震颤抖动,要求每秒颤动 10 次左右为宜。颤法与"动"分不开,所以又叫它颤动手法。将大拇指垂直地点在患者痛点,全腕用力颤动,带动拇指产生震颤性地抖动,叫单指颤动法。用拇指与示指,或示指与中指,放在患者痛处或眉头等处,利用腕力进行颤动叫双指颤动法。

（三）按

用手拇指螺纹面或者把两手掌叠起,逐渐用力下压,有节奏地按压。在临床上有指按法和掌按法之分,按法亦可与其他手法结合,如果与压法结合则为按压法。若与揉法结合,则为按揉法。

（四）揉

用手指或是手掌贴近皮肤进行旋转活动。用大鱼际、掌根,或手指螺纹面吸附于一定的治疗部位,做轻柔缓和的环旋运动,并带动该部位的皮下组织,称之为揉法。以大鱼际为力点,称鱼际揉法;揉法具有消瘀去积,调和血行的作用,对于局部痛点,使用揉法十分合适。

（五）拿

用一手或两手拿住皮肤、肌肉或筋膜,用力向上紧缩捏拿起来,随后放下。拿法是推拿常用手法之一,在临床上有三指拿(拇指与示、中指相对用力)和五指拿(拇指与其余四指相对用力)之分。

（六）摩

用手指或手掌给予柔软的往返抚摩。用手指或手掌在患者身体的适当部位,给以柔软的抚摩。摩法多配合按法和推法,有常用于上肢和肩端的单手摩法和常用于胸部的双手摩法。摩法的动作与揉法有相似之处,但摩法用力更轻,仅在体表抚摩;而揉法用力略沉,手法要带动皮下组织。

（七）捏

在适当部位,利用手指把皮肤和肌肉从骨面上捏起来,同时用手指把皮肤和肌肉捏紧,然后轻轻放松,如此连续交替。捏法和拿法有某些类似之处,但是拿法要用手的全力,捏法则着重在手指上。拿法用力要重些,捏法用力要轻些。

（八）推

手指或手掌用力向前或向上、向外推动,推挤肌肉。推法在成人推拿里的应用主要是平推法。在小儿推拿里的应用有直推、分推、旋推等多种方法。

四、推拿适应证(Indications of *Tuina*)

1.各种疼痛性疾病　偏头痛,前、后头痛,三叉神经痛,肋间神经痛,股神经痛,坐骨神经痛,腰背神经痛,四肢关节痛(包括肩、肘、腕、膝、踝、指或趾关节疼痛),因风湿而引起的如肩、背、腰、膝等部的肌肉疼痛等。

2.各种炎症性疾病　急性或慢性风湿性关节炎、退行性脊柱炎、膝关节骨关节炎、关节滑囊肿痛和关节强直等。

3.内科疾病　感冒、头痛、失眠、胃脘痛、胃下垂、呃逆、便秘、慢性泄泻、腰痛、遗尿、痹证、偏瘫等。

4.妇科疾病　月经不调、痛经、闭经、慢性盆腔炎、乳腺炎、产后耻骨联合分离症等。

5.儿科疾病　婴幼儿腹泻、小儿营养不良、小儿遗尿、小儿肌性斜颈、小儿疳积、小儿急慢惊风、小儿麻痹症后遗症等。

6.其他　美容、减肥、保健养生、休闲放松、娱乐等。

五、推拿禁忌证(Contraindications of *Tuina*)

1.诊断不明的急性脊髓损伤或伴有脊髓症状的患者,在未排除脊椎骨折时切忌推拿。出现脑脊髓症状时须排除蛛网膜下腔出血,这也是推拿禁忌证。

2. 各种骨折、骨关节结核、骨髓炎、骨肿瘤、严重的老年性骨质疏松症患者,推拿可能引起病理性骨折、肿瘤扩散转移或炎症发展扩散。因此也属于推拿禁忌证。

3. 严重的心、肺、肝、肾功能衰竭的患者或身体过于虚弱者,由于不能承受强刺激,因此一般不宜接受推拿治疗。

4. 各种急性传染病,急性腹膜炎包括胃、十二指肠溃疡穿孔者,禁忌推拿治疗,应考虑手术剖腹探查。

5. 有出血倾向或有血液病的患者,推拿可能引起局部皮下出血,故不宜推拿治疗。

6. 避免在有皮肤损伤的部位施手法。但在有压疮的周围施轻手法改善局部血液循环,可使缺血性坏死的创面逐渐愈合。

7. 妊娠 3 个月以上的妇女的腹部、臀部、腰骶部,为了防止流产,不宜在这些部位施手法。

8. 精神病患者或精神过度紧张时不宜推拿治疗。

六、推拿注意事项(Precautions of *Tuina*)

1. 按摩前要修整指甲、热水洗手,同时,将指环等有碍操作的物品,预先摘掉。

2. 操作过程中要认真、严肃、注意力集中,随时观察患者对手法的反应,若有不适,应及时进行调整,以防发生意外事故。态度要和蔼,严肃细心,要耐心地向患者解释病情,争取患者合作。

3. 患者与操作者的位置要安排合适;特别是患者坐卧等姿势,要舒适而又便于操作。

4. 按摩手法一定要先轻后重,由浅入深,循序渐进,使体表有个适应的过程,切勿用力过大,以免擦伤皮肤;同时还要注意双手清洁,勤剪指甲,讲究手部卫生,并且要保持双手有一定的温度。并随时观察患者表情,使患者有舒服感。

5. 按摩时间每次以 20~30 分钟为宜,按摩次数以 10~15 次为宜,疗程间宜休息 2~3 日。

6. 患者在大怒、大喜、大恐、大悲等情绪激动的情况下,不要立即按摩。

7. 对于过饱、酒后及大量运动后的患者,一般不予立即施以推拿治疗。

8. 按摩时,有些患者容易入睡,除少数直接接触皮肤的手法(如擦法、推法等)外,治疗时要用按摩巾覆盖治疗部位以防着凉,注意室温。当风之处,不要按摩。小儿推拿多使用介质,以保护皮肤。

Tuina refers to a method for health care and disease treatment by applying specific operating manipulation or limb activities on meridians, acupoints and certain parts of the human body.

Also known as *anmo*, *qiaomo* and massage.

It has the functions of dredging meridians, facilitating joints, promoting the circulation of *qi* and blood, adjusting viscera functions, enhancing the disease resistance of human body and achieving the purpose of disease treatment and prevention, which is widely used in clinical departments.

"Pushing" and "Grasping" are the most commonly used and representative manipulations in massage. Manipulations and *Gongfa* are important contents and main therapeutic techniques of massage.

In addition to health care, weight loss, beauty care and fatigue elimination, massage therapy is also widely used in the clinical treatment of many diseases in the departments of spine surgery, orthopedics, internal medicine, gynecology, pediatrics and ENT.

People habitually call those used for medical treatment "*Tuina*", those used for health care "*Anmo*", while traditional Chinese medicine collectively calls them "*Tuina*".

Tuina is the oldest art of mankind, which originated in ancient times and has a long history. It is a bright pearl in traditional Chinese medicine. *Tuina* originated from the self-protection of human.

In ancient times, human beings often suffered from bruises and pains during hard work. And when there was discomfort in certain parts of the body, people would touch and press there unconsciously, and the pain would be relieved, so they gradually formed an understanding of massage. After thousands of repetition, ancient people realized that they could relieve or eliminate pains by acting on certain parts in a suitable way of compression, so they gradually applied it to daily activities and medical behavior, resulting in the original *tuina*.

During the Qin, Jin, and Han dynasties, *tuina* therapy got rid of the shackles of empirical medicine and became a subject with national characteristics and theoretical foundation, occupying an important position in traditional Chinese medicine.

1 Principle of *Tuina*

In fact, *tuina* is to act on the surface of the human body through different techniques, to achieve the balance between various viscera and corresponding tissues through meridians and acupoints. It can accelerate the metabolism of the body, and repair all kinds of physical injuries so as to adjust the physiological and pathological state of the human body, realizing the function of disease treatment and health care.

The principle of *tuina* is closely related to manipulations, and its theoretical basis is the meridian theory of traditional Chinese medicine.

It can also correct anatomical abnormalities through external force, especially joint dislocation, tendon subluxation and other diseases caused by anatomical abnormalities.

2　Function of *Tuina*

The main function of *tuina* is to relieve people's tension and pain.

It can make *qi* and blood run normally, improve blood circulation, dredge meridians, and reduce the pain of the body.

2.1　Dreding Meridians and Harmonizing *Qi* and Blood

Qi is the commander of blood and blood is the mother of *qi*. Only when *qi* moves normally can blood circulation functions well. Stagnation of *qi* causes stasis of blood and vice versa. Massage manipulations act on the meridians and collaterals on the body surface, generating local reactions and playing the role of stimulating and adjusting the meridian *qi*.

By regulating the *qi* movement, and promoting blood circulation for removing obstruction in collalera, it adjusts appropriately the internal disorder so as to make the blood channel unobstructed and the securith function of *qi* to be normal, thus playing a positive therapeutic role.

Huangdi Neijing (*Yellow Emperor's Canon of Medicine*) says: "The disease due to stagnation of the channels and collaterals and can be cured by *tuina* (massage). " This shows that *tuina* has the effect of dredging meridians.

From a physiological point of view, it has a certain stimulation to the body by massaging the body surface.

By stimulating the peripheral nerves, promoting the blood and lymph circulation and the metabolic process between the tissues, the functions of tissues and organs can be coordinated, and the metabolic level of functions can be improved.

2.2　Releasing the Channel Sinews and Relieving Swelling and Pain

Most of the diseases treated by *tuina* are the symptoms of contusion. *Tuina* is operated on the meridians and acupoints in the local and distant parts of the lesion by means of traction, flexion, pushing, pressing, pulling and shaking. It can repair the injury, restore the dislocation or dislocation, correct the dislocation and spondylolisthesis, and play the role of regulating tendons, reducing swelling and relieving pain, thereby playing the role of releasing and relaxing the channel sinews, reducing swelling and relieving pain, and restoring the normal living and movement functions of the human body.

2.3　Dispelling Cold and Removing *Bi*-impediment, Lubricating and Facilitating the Joints

It is recorded in *Bi Lun of Su Wen* (*Discussion on Bi-Syndrome* the chapter of *Plain Conversation*): "The interaction of wind, cold and dampness causes *Bi* (stagnation or obstruction). If wind is in predomination, it causes *Xingbi* (Migratory–Stagnation), if cold is in predomination, it causes *Tongbi* (Pain–Stagnation), and if dampness is in predomination, it causes *Zhuobi* (Heavy–Stagnation). *Bi*–Sydrome in the bones leads to heaviness of the body, *Bi*–Syndrome in the Channels leads tounsmooth flow of blood, *Bi*–Syndrome in the sinews leads to inflexibility of the limbs, *Bi*–Syndrome in the muscles leads tonumbness, and *Bi*–Syndrome in the skin leads to cold. "

Massage has the functions of relaxing tendons and removing obstruction in collaterals, lubricating and facilitating joints, regulating blood circulation and removing pain of *Bi*–impediment disorders.

Wind–cold–dampness impediment obstructs meridians, hinders the movement of *qi* and blood, resulting in soreness and numbness in muscle, tendons, bones and joint, heaviness of the body or joint swelling, deformation, movement disorders, and even abnormal viscera function.

Tuina plays a role in loosening adhesion and facilitating joints that are stuck and rigid by massage manipulations. It can improve local nutrition supply and promote metabolism for those with local soft tissue degeneration, thereby gradually improving or restoring the denatured tissue.

3 Basic Manipulations of *Tuina*

The manipulations of *tuina* are various and inconsistent. They are not simply used in isolation but often cooperate with each other, requiring them to be lasting, forceful and balanced. To sum up, there are eight basic manipulations used in tuina.

3.1 Tapping

A manipulation to tap the area to be treated with finger, palm or a hollow fist. The strength of the hand should be accurate, soft and flexible. The right technique can give the patient a sense of ease, otherwise it is not appropriate. The time is about 1–2 minutes or 3 minutes. In very few cases, time can be extended or shortened according to the condition of disease. This manipulation can also be carried out after massage, or it can be mixed with other massage manipulations.

3.2 Vibrating

A manipulation to slightly shake the fingertips or palm. It is appropriate to vibrate about 10 times per second. Single–finger vibrating is to place the thumb vertically at the pain point of the patient, and vibrate the whole wrist forcefully todrive the thumb to tremble. Double–finger vibrating is to use the thumb and index finger, or index finger and middle finger to vibrate on the patient's pain part or eyebrow.

3.3　Pressing

A manipulation to apply perpendicular pressure to the surface of the body with the palmar side of the fingers or palms. In clinic, it can be divided into finger pressing and palm pressing. It can also be combined with other manipulations such as forceful pressing manipulation and kneading manipulation.

3.4　Kneading

A manipulation to apply perpendicular pressure to the surface of the body with the fingers or palms. Kneading is a manipulation to using the great thenar, palm root, or the palmar side of the fingers to attach to a certain treatment area, do a gentle circular movement, and drive the subcutaneous tissue of the area. Thenar-kneading manipulation is to knead and exert force on the area to be treated with the great thenar. Kneading has the effects of eliminating stasis and removing accumulation, harmonizing blood flow. And for local pain points, the use of kneading method is very suitable.

3.5　Grasping

A manipulation to pinch and knead the skin, muscle or anadesma to be treated with the one hand or two hands. It is one of the commonly used massage manipulations, which can be divided into three-finger grasping (use thumb, index and middle finger) and five-finger grasping (use five fingers).

3.6　Circular Rubbing

A manipulation to softly rub the area to be treated circularly with the fingers or palms. It is often combined with pressing and pushing. There are one-handed circular rubbing commonly used for upper limbs and shoulders, and two-handed circular rubbing commonly used for chest. The actions of circular rubbing is similar to that of kneading, but the force used in circular rubbing is lighter, only caressing on the body surface, while the force of kneading is slightly heavier, the pressure is supposed to reach subcutaneous tissues.

3.7　Pinching

A manipulation to apply coordinated pressure to the area to be treated with the fingers. Use fingers to pinch the skin and muscles from the bone surface at the proper place. There are some similarities between pinching and grasping. But grassping requires the full strength of the hand, and pinching focuses on the fingers. The strength of grasping should be heavier than pinching.

3.8　Pushing

Pushing is to push the fingers or palms forward or upward or outward to squeeze the muscles. The application of pushing manipulation in adult is mainly flat pushing. And there are many methods used in pediatric *tuina*, such as flate pushing, forked pushing, spin pushing and so on.

4　Indications of *Tuina*

4.1　Painful Diseases

Migraine headache, headache at the front and back, neuralgia at the trident, neuralgia at the rib, neuralgia at the thigh, neuralgia at the sciatica, neuralgia at the waist and back, pain at the joints of the limbs (including pain at the shoulders, elbows, wrists, knees, ankles, fingers, toes joints), caused by rheumatism such as muscle pain at the shoulders, back, waist, knees, etc.

4.2　Inflammatory Diseases

Acute or chronic rheumatoid arthritis, degenerative spondylitis, knee osteoarthritis, joint landslide pain and joint ankylosis, etc.

4.3　Internal Medical Diseases

Cold, headache, insomnia, stomachache, gastroptosis, hiccup, constipation, chronic diarrhea, lumbago, enuresis, *Bi*-impediment and paralysis, etc.

4.4　Gynecologic Diseases

Menstrual irregularity amenorrhea, amenorrhea, chronic pelvic inflammation, mastitis and postpartum pubescent union separation, etc.

4.5　Pediatric Diseases

Infantile diarrhea, infantile malnutrition, infantile enuresis, infantile muscular torticollis, infantile amalgamation, sudden and slow convulsions, polio sequelae, etc.

4.6　Other

Beauty care, weight loss, health care, leisure and relaxation, entertainment, etc.

5　Contraindications of *Tuina*

5.1　It's not advised to apply massage to patients with acute spinal cord injury of unknown diagnosis or with spinal cord symptoms should not be treated with massage when vertebral fracture has not been ruled out. Massage is contraindicated in patients with encephalomyelitis because subarachnoid hemorrhage must be excluded.

5.2　It's not advised to apply massage to patients with fractures, bone joint tuberculosis, myelitis, bone tumors, and severe senile osteoporosis, for it may cause pathological fracture, tumor diffusion and metastasis, or inflammation development and diffusion.

5.3　It's not advised to apply massage to patients with severe heart, lung, liver and kidney failure or those who are too weak to bear strong stimulation.

5.4　It's not advised to apply massage to patients with various acute infectious diseases, acute peritonitis including gastric and duodenal ulcer perforation. Abdominal exploration surgery can be considered.

5.5　It's not advised to apply massage to patients with hemorrhagic disease because massage may cause local subcutaneous hemorrhage.

5.6　Generally, massage is avoided in areas with skin damage. But applying a gentle manipulation to improve local blood circulation around the bedsores can make the wound of ischemic necrosis gradually heal.

5.7　In order to prevent abortion, the abdomen, buttocks and lumbosacral parts of women who are pregnant for more than 3 months should not be manipulated.

5.8　It is forbidden to use massage to patients with mental illness or excessive mental tension.

6　Precautions of *Tuina*

6.1　Manicure your nails and wash your hands with hot water before massage and remove rings and other items that may hinder operation.

6.2　Be careful, serious and focused in the process of operation. Always observe the patient's reaction to the manipulation, if there is discomfort, timely adjustment should be made to prevent accidents. Be kind, serious and careful. Explain the illness to the patient patiently, and strive for patient cooperation.

6.3　The position of the patient and the operator should be arranged appropriately.

In particular, the sitting and lying posture of the patient should be comfortable and convenient to operate.

6.4　The manipulations must be light first and then heavy, from shallow to deep, step by step, so that the body surface has an adaptation process. Avoid force that may scratch the skin. Pay attention to the cleanliness of hands and nails, and keep hands at a certain temperature. Observing the expression of patient at any time so as to make the patient feel comfortable.

6.5　Massage duration should be 20-30 minutes each time, 10-15 times every course, and rest for 2−3 days in the course of treatment.

6.6　Patients should not massage immediately in cases of great anger,joy,fear,grief and other emotional excitement.

6.7　It is not advised to apply massage immediately to people who are over−eating,drunk and exercised.

6.8　When massaging,some patients are easy to fall asleep. Except for a few methods that directly touch the skin（such as rubbing and pushing）,towels should be used to cover the treatment area to prevent colds. Pay attention to room temperature,don't massage when feel the wind. Infantile massage need more media to protect the skin.

第二节　艾　灸
（Moxibustion）

艾灸,别称灸疗或灸法,是用艾叶制成的艾条、艾炷,产生艾热,借助热力和药物的作用刺激人体穴位或特定部位,通过激发经气的活动来调整人体紊乱的生理生化功能,从而达到防病治病目的的一种治疗方法。艾灸作用机制与针灸有相近之处,并与针灸有相辅相成的治疗作用,具有操作简单、成本低廉、效果显著等诸多优点。

一、艾灸原理（Principle of Moxibustion）

（一）局部刺激作用

艾灸具有温煦作用,对人体局部起到温热刺激,具有较强的渗透力,使毛细血管扩张,能增强局部血液循环和淋巴循环,皮肤组织的代谢能力也会得到加强,促进炎症、粘连、渗出物、血肿等病理产物的吸收。局部温热刺激还可以降低神经系统的兴奋性,从而达到镇静、止痛的作用。温热还能促进药物的吸收,将艾绒本身的药效、艾条中其他添加药材以及间隔物的药效充分发挥出来。

（二）经络调节作用

经络学说是灸疗的基础理论,对穴位的刺激作用最终会通过人体经络系统对人体五脏六腑、四肢起到调节作用,使人的整体功能保持良好运转。灸疗法的刺激,通过经络传递调节,激发出机体出现相互协同的效果,产生生理上的放大叠加效果和作用,最终使疾病痊愈。

（三）免疫功能调节作用

人体免疫力就是人体对病原体或毒素所具备的抵抗力,临床研究证明,艾灸疗法能激活皮肤中某些酶类参与机体的免疫调节,增加白细胞的吞噬功能,提高免疫效应,增强人体免疫功能。

二、艾灸作用（Function of Moxibustion）

（一）温经散寒

艾灸正是应用其温热刺激，起到温经通痹的作用。气血的运行，遇温则散，遇寒则凝。通过热灸对经络穴位的温热性刺激，可以温经散寒，加强机体气血运行，达到临床治疗目的。灸法可用于血寒运行不畅，留滞凝涩引起的痹证、腹泻等疾病。

（二）行气通络

经络分布于人体各部，内联脏腑，外布体表肌肉、骨骼等组织。正常的机体，气血在经络中周流不息，循序运行。因为"六淫"的侵袭，人体局部容易气血凝滞，经络受阻，出现肿胀疼痛等症状或一系列功能障碍。艾灸相应的穴位，就可起到疏通经络、调和气血、平衡功能的作用，以及增强人体抗病的作用。

（三）扶阳固脱

阳气是人体健康的根本，人的寿命也跟阳气是否健旺有关。阳病则阴盛，阴盛则为寒、为厥，甚至元气虚陷，脉微欲脱。由于艾叶有纯阳的性质，再加上火本属阳，两阳相得，往往可以起到扶阳固脱、回阳救逆、挽救垂危之疾的作用，在临床上常用于中风脱症、急性腹痛吐泻、痢疾等急症的急救。

（四）升阳举陷

阳气虚弱不固可致上虚下实，气虚下陷，出现脱肛、阴挺、崩漏、久泄久痢、滑胎等症。艾灸不仅可以起到益气温阳、升阳举陷、安胎固经等作用，对卫阳不固、腠理疏松者亦有效果，使机体功能恢复正常。

（五）拔毒泄热

艾灸能以热引热，使热外出。艾灸既能散寒，又能清热，对机体原来的功能状态起双向调节作用。

三、常用艾灸法（Commen Moxibustion Methods）

（一）艾炷灸

用艾绒或药艾制成圆柱形的艾炷，将艾炷放在腧穴上施灸。可分为直接灸和间接灸。

1.直接灸　又名着肤灸，是将大小适宜的艾炷，直接放在皮肤上施灸。直接灸因施灸目的和对皮肤刺激程度的不同，又分为瘢痕灸、无瘢痕灸和发疱灸3种。

（1）瘢痕灸：又名化脓灸，施灸时需将皮肤烧伤化脓，愈后留有瘢痕。用黄豆或枣核大小的艾炷,直接置于穴位上施灸,局部组织经烫伤后化脓、结痂,痂脱落后留有永久性的瘢痕,故名瘢痕灸。施灸时由于火烧灼皮肤,因此可产生剧痛,此时可用手在施灸腧穴周围轻轻拍打,借以缓解疼痛。正常情况下,灸后1周左右,施灸部位化脓形成灸疮,5~6周,灸疮自行痊愈,结痂脱落后留下瘢痕。临床上常用于治疗哮喘、肺结核、瘰疬、慢性胃肠病等慢性疾病。

（2）无瘢痕灸:又称非化脓灸,施灸以温熨为度,不起疱,多用小艾炷。因其皮肤无灼伤,故灸后不化脓,不留瘢痕。此法适用于慢性虚寒性疾患,如哮喘、风寒湿痹等。

（3）发疱灸:临床上多用小艾炷,对皮肤的灼烫程度较轻。发疱灸适用于一般慢性虚寒性疾病,如哮喘、眩晕、慢性腹泻、皮肤疣等。

2.间接灸　又称间隔灸、隔物灸。是用某种物品将艾炷与施灸腧穴部位的皮肤隔开,进行施灸的方法。所隔的物品常用生姜、大蒜、盐、附子片等。

（1）隔姜灸:是用鲜姜切成直径2~3厘米、厚0.2~0.3厘米的薄片,中间以针刺数孔,然后将姜片置于应灸的腧穴部位或患处,再将艾炷放在姜片上点燃施灸。具有温胃止吐、散寒止痛的功效。

（2）隔蒜灸:是用鲜大蒜头,切成厚0.2~0.3厘米的薄片,中间以针刺数孔,然后置于应灸腧穴或患处,然后将艾炷放在蒜片上,点燃施灸。具有清热解毒、杀虫等功效。

（3）隔盐灸:是用干燥纯净的食盐填敷于脐部,或于盐上再置一薄姜片,上置大艾炷施灸。具有回阳、救逆、固脱之力。

（4）隔附子饼灸:是将附子研成粉末,用酒调和做成直径约3厘米、厚0.2~0.5厘米的附子饼,中间以针刺数孔,放在应灸腧穴或患处,上面再放艾炷施灸,直到灸完所规定壮数为止,具有温阳补肾等作用。

（二）艾条灸

艾条灸是将艾绒或药艾制成圆筒状长条形艾卷,然后点燃进行施灸。常用的施灸方法有温和灸和雀啄灸。

1.温和灸　施灸时将艾条对准应灸的腧穴部位或患处,距皮肤3~5厘米,熏烤使患者局部有温热感而无灼痛为宜。

2.雀啄灸　施灸时艾条与施灸部位的皮肤并不固定在一定距离,而是像鸟雀啄食一样,一上一下活动地施灸。另外也可均匀地上、下或向左、右方向移动或做反复的旋转施灸。

（三）温针灸

温针灸又称温针疗法,是针刺与艾灸结合应用的一种方法,适用于既需要留针而又适宜用艾灸的病症。操作时,将针刺入腧穴得气后,用一段长约2厘米左右的艾条,插在针柄上,点燃施灸。待艾绒或艾条烧完后,除去灰烬,出针。

四、艾灸适应证（Indications of Moxibustion）

1. 寒凝血滞、经络痹阻引起的各种病症，如风寒湿痹、痛经、经闭、寒疝腹痛等。

2. 外感风寒之表证及中焦虚寒呕吐、腹痛、泄泻等。

3. 脾肾阳虚，元气暴脱之证，如久泄、久痢、遗尿、遗精、阳痿、早泄、虚脱、休克等。

4. 中气不足、气虚下陷、脏器下垂之证，如胃下垂、肾下垂、子宫脱垂、脱肛等。

5. 外科疮疡初起，以及疮疡溃久不愈，有促进愈合、生肌长肉的作用。

6. 用于治疗气逆上冲的病证，如脚气冲心、肝阳上升之证可灸涌泉治之。

7. 阴虚热证如喉痹、肺痨等。

8. 防病保健。

五、艾灸禁忌证（Contraindications of Moxibustion）

1. 暴露在外的部位，如颜面部，不用直接灸法，以防形成瘢痕，影响美观。

2. 大动脉处、心脏部位、静脉血管、肌腱潜在部位，妊娠妇女的腰骶部、下腹部以及乳头，阴部、睾丸等处均不宜施灸。

3. 患有重病、急性传染性疾病者，严重心血管疾病伴有心功能不全者，严重贫血症患者，精神分裂症患者，有明显出血性疾病等患者，均不宜艾灸。

4. 高热、昏迷、抽搐期间的患者，或身体极度衰竭、形体太过消瘦的患者不宜施灸。

5. 皮肤过敏严重者的患处，以及过饥过饱、大汗淋漓、醉酒、身体极度疲劳不宜进行灸疗。

6. 做过植入性手术（如心脏起搏器或金属）者、大血管处、严重糖尿病患者要慎灸。

7. 精神病等无自制能力的患者忌用灸法。

六、艾灸注意事项（Precautions of Moxibustion）

1. 施灸时要注意思想集中，专心致志，不要在施灸时分散注意力，以免艾条移动，烫伤皮肤，并且注意防火。

2. 要注意体位舒适、自然、便于操作，找准穴位，以保证艾灸的效果。

3. 要注意保暖，因施灸时要暴露部分体表部位，在冬季更要保暖。

4. 初次使用灸法要注意掌握好刺激量，从小剂量开始，循序渐进。如用小艾炷，或灸的时间短一些，壮数少一些，以后再逐渐加大剂量。

5. 注意施灸的时间，如失眠症要在临睡前施灸。不要饭前空腹时和在饭后立即施灸。

6. 操作过程中注意观察患者，防止晕灸，晕灸会出现头晕、眼花、恶心、面色苍白、心慌、汗出等症状，严重者甚至会发生晕倒。出现晕灸后，要立即停灸，并躺下静卧。

7. 注意施灸温度的调节,对于糖尿病、肢体麻木、皮肤感觉迟钝者或小儿,应注意调节施灸温度,防止烫伤。

8. 要防止感染,如果施灸部位出现水疱,小的无须处理。大的用碘伏棉球消毒后,用一次性注射器抽吸,再用无菌纱布包扎。

Moxibustion, also known as moxibustion therapy, is a method of treating moxa strips and moxa columns made of moxa leaves, which generates moxa heat, stimulates acupoints or specific parts of the human body with the help of heat and medicine. It can adjust the physiological and biochemical functions of human body disorders by stimulating the activities of meridians and *qi*, so as to achieve the purpose of preventing and treating diseases.

The moxibustion action mechanism is similar to acupuncture and has complementary therapeutic effects with acupuncture. It has the advantages of simple operation, low costs and obvious effects.

1 Principle of Moxibustion

1.1 Local Stimulation

The moxibustion has the function of warming and stimulating. It has strong penetrability to local human body, causes capillary blood vessels to expand. It can enhance local blood circulation and lymphatic circulation, strengthen the metabolic ability of skin tissue, and promote the absorption of pathological products such as inflammation, adhesion, exudate and hematoma.

Local warm stimulation can also reduce the excitability of the nervous system, thereby achieving the effects of sedation and analgesia.

Warm can also promote the absorption of medicines, and fully exert the medicinal effects of the moxa velvet itself, other medicinal materials added to the moxa strips and the medicinal effects of the spacers.

1.2 Regulating Meridians

The theory of meridians is the basic theory of moxibustion. The stimulation effects on acupoints will eventually play a role in regulating the five *zang* organs, six *fu* organs and four limbs of the human body through the meridian system of the human body, so that the overall function of the human body can maintain good operation. The stimulation of the moxibustion is regulated through meridians.

It stimulates the synergistic effect of the body, produces a physiological magnifying and superposition effect, and finally makes the disease cured.

1.3 Regulating Immunization

Human immunity is the resistance of human body to pathogens or toxins. Clinical studies have proved that moxibustion can activate some enzymes in skin to participate in immune regulation, increase phagocytosis of leukocytes, improve immune effect and enhance human immune function.

2　Function of Moxibustion

2.1　Warming Meridians for Dispelling Cold

Through warm stimulation, moxibustion serves to warm meridians and dredging *Bi*-impediment disorders. The movement of *qi* and bloodis scattered when it is warm, and condensed when it is cold. Through the warm stimulation of meridians and acupoints by moxibustion, it can warm meridians and dispel cold, strengthen the circulation of *qi* and blood, and achieve the purpose of clinical treatment. Moxibustion can be used for diseases such as impediment and diarrhea caused by poor blood circulation and astringency.

2.2　Circulating *Qi* and Unblocking Collaterals

The meridians and collaterals are distributed in all parts of the human body, which are internally connected to the viscera, and to the muscles, bones and other tissues on the external surface. In a normal organism, *qi* and blood flow around in the meridians and run in an orderly manner. Because of the invasion of "six excesses", the local body is prone to *qi* and blood stagnation, obstruction of meridians, swelling and pain or a series of functional disorders. Moxibustion at the corresponding acupoints can dredge meridians and collaterals, reconcile *qi* and blood, balance the function of the body, and enhance the ability of disease resistance of the human body.

2.3　Strengthening *Yang* to Prevent Collapse

Yangqi is the foundation of human health, and people's life span is also related to it. *Yang* diseases are mainly caused by the excess of *yin*, and the excess of yin causes cold, syncope, or even the deficiency of *Yuan*-primordial *qi*, and pulse desertion disease.

Because the moxa leaves have the nature of pure *yang*, and fire pertains to *yang*, it can often play the role of strengthening *yang* to prevent collapse, restoring *yang* and rescuing patient from collapse and saving dying patients in clinic, it is often used in the first aid of stroke, acute abdominal pain, diarrhea, dysentery and other emergencies.

2.4　Reinforcing *Yang* to lift Sinking *Qi*

The deficiency of *yangqi* can lead to upperr deficiency and lower excess, deficiency of *qi*, sinking of *qi*, and the symptoms such as anal detachment, *yin* stiffening, collapse, chronic diarrhea and dysentery and tire slipping.

Moxibustion can not only play the roles of invigorating *qi* and warming *yang*, reinforce *yang to lift sinking qi*, preventing miscariage and securing meridians, but also has the effect on those who are not firm in defending the *yang* and are loose in purgatory and restore the function of the body to normal.

2.5 Removing Toxin and Relieving Heat

Moxibustion can draw heat by heat and make the heat go out. Moxibustion not only dispels cold, but also clears heat, and plays a two-way role in regulating the original functional state of the body.

3　Common Moxibustion Methods

3.1 Moxa Cone Moxibustion

A method to place a moxa cone made by moxa wool or medicinal moxa to the selected acupoint and then ignite. It can be divided into direct and indirect moxibustion.

（1）Direct moxibustion, also known as skin moxibustion, is to put moxa cone of a suitable size directly on the skin for moxibustion.

Direct moxibustion is divided into three categories: scarring moxibustion, non − scarring moxibustion and vesiculating moxibustion according to the purpose of moxibustion and the degree of skin irritation.

1）Scarring moxibustion, also known as suppurative moxibustion, It may burn and purify the skin during moxibustion, and leave scars after it heals.

Moxibustion is applied directly on the acupuncture point with a moxa cone of the size of a soybean or a date palm, and the local tissues become septic and scabbed after the burn, leaving a permanent scar after the scab falls off, hence the name scarring moxibustion.

During moxibustion, the skin can be burned by fire, so severe pain can be generated. At this time, the hand can be gently patted around the moxibustion acupoint to relieve the pain.

Under normal circumstances, about one week after moxibustion, the moxibustion site festers pus to form moxibustion sore, and about 5−6 weeks later, it healsautomatically, leaving scars after scabs fall off.

Clinically, it is often used to treat chronic diseases such as asthma, pulmonary tuberculosis, chronic gastroenteropathy.

2）Non−scarring moxibustion, also known as non−suppurative moxibustion, is a method to apply burning moxa on the body and remove it before the skin burns enough to scar. It uses small moxa cone more.

Because there is no burns on the skin,there is no pus and no scars after moxibustion.

The method is applicable to chronic deficiency and cold diseases,such as asthma and wind-cold-dampness impediment.

3)Vesiculating moxibustion Small moxa is often used in Vesiculating moxibustion,and the scalding degree of skin is lighter.

It is applicable to common chronic deficiency and cold diseases,such as asthma, dizziness,chronic diarrhea,skin warts.

(2)Indirect moxibustion,also known as insulated moxibustion,It is a method to place some insulated materials between the moxa cone and the skin. Ginger,garlic,salt,aconite are the common insulated materials.

1)Ginger-Insulated Moxibustion:Cut fresh ginger into thin slices with the diameter of 2- 3 cm and the thickness of 0.2-0.3 cm,and then prick a plurality of holes in the middle,then place the ginger slices on the acupoints or affected parts of the moxibustion,and then put the moxa on the ginger slices for lighting and moxibustion.

It has the effects of warming stomach and relieving vomiting,dispelling cold and relieving pain.

2)Garlic-Insulated Moxibustion:Cut fresh garlic into thin slices with thickness of 0.2- 0.3 cm for garlic separation,prick several holes in the middle of garlic separation,then place it in the acupoint or affected place for moxibustion,and put the moxa on the garlic slices and light it.

It has the effects of clearing heat and detoxification,killing insects and so on.

3)Salt-Insulated Moxibustion:Apply dry,pure salt to the umbilicus,or place a thin slice of ginger on top of the salt and apply moxibustion with a large moxa cone. It has the effects of resuscitating yang and preventing collapsen.

4)Monkshood Cake - Insulated Moxibustiong: Grinding aconite into powder through aconite cake moxibustion,mixing it with wine to prepare monkshood cake with the diameter of about 3 cm and the thickness of about 0.2-0.5 cm. With several holes pierced by needles in the middle,placed on the acupuncture point or the affected area,and moxibustion is applied with moxa cones on top until the required number is completed,which has the effect of warming the *yang* and tonifying the kidney.

3.2　Moxa stick moxibustion

Moxa stick moxibustion is to make moxa wool or medicinal moxa into a cylindrical strip- shaped moxa roll,and then light it for moxibustion.

Common moxibustion methods are gentle moxibustion and Sparrow-pecking moxibustion.

（1）Gentle Moxibustion：A method to keep the end of an ignited moxa stick at a fixed distance（3-5 cm）from the selected area until patients feel warm without burning pain.

（2）Sparrow-Pecking Moxibustion：A method to place an ignited moxa stick near the moxibustion area flexibly and to move it up and down like a pecking bird.

In addition, it can be uniformly moved upwards and downwards or in the left and right directions or rotated repeatedly.

3.3　Needle-warming Moxibustion

Needle-warming moxibustion, also called warm acupuncture therapy, is a combination of acupuncture and moxibustion, suitable for both needle retention and symptoms suitable for treating by moxibustion.

When operating, after the needle is pricked into the acupoint to get *qi*, use a section of moxa strips with the length of about 2 cm inserted on the needle handle and ignited for moxibustion.

When the moxa wool or the moxa stick is burnt, remove the ash and take out the needle.

4　Indications of Moxibustion

（1）Diseases caused by blood stasis due to cold coagulation and obstruction of meridians and collaterals, such as Wind-cold-dampness impediment, dysmenorrhea, amenorrhea, cold hernia, abdominal pain.

（2）Wind cold exterior pattern and vomiting, abdominal pain, diarrhea due to deficiency cold of middle *jiao*.

（3）*Yang* deficiency of the spleen and kidney, and pattern of sudden collapse of *Yuan*-primordial *qi*, such as chronic ejaculation, chronic dysentery, enuresis, ejaculation, impotence of yang, premature ejaculation, collapse and shock.

（4）Deficiency and sinking pattern of middle *qi*, and ptosis of organs such as gastroptosis, nephroptosis, uterine detachment, anal detachment.

（5）Surgical sores at the beginning, and sores that do not heal for a long time. It has the effects of promoting healing and the growth of muscle and flesh.

（6）*Qi* counter-flow pattern. For example, patterns of weak foot affecting heart and hyperactivity of liver *yang* can be cured by moxibustion on *Yongquan*（KI1）.

（7）Kidney *yin* deficiency pattern such as throat impediment and phthisis.

（8）Disease prevention and health care.

5　Contraindications of Moxibustion

（1）It is not advised to use direct moxibustion on exposure parts such as face lest scar be formed to affect beauty.

(2) It is not advised to use moxibustion on the areas including the aortas, heart, veins and tendons, lumbosacral region and lower abdomen of pregnant women, nipple, genitals and testis.

(3) It is not advised to apply moxibustion to people with serious illness, acute infectious diseases, severe cardiovascular diseases with cardiac insufficiency, severe anemia, schizophrenia and obvious hemorrhagic diseases.

(4) It is not advised to apply moxibustion to patients with high fever, coma and convulsions, or people in failure or emaciated condition.

(5) It is not advised to apply moxibustion to people who are famished, over-eating, sweating, drunk and over-fatigue. And it should not be applied to the affected part of patients with severe skin allergy.

(6) It is not advised to apply moxibustion to people who have undergone implantation surgery (implanting cardiac pacemaker or metal in the body) and those who with severe diabetes should use moxibustion with caution.

(7) It is forbidden to use moxibustion to patients with mental illness.

6　Precautions of Moxibustion

(1) When applying moxibustion, focus the mind and do not distract attention lest the movement of moxa sticks scald skin, and prevent fire.

(2) A comfortable and easy-for-operation position ensures the effect of moxibustion.

(3) Keep warm, because some parts of the body should be exposed when moxibustion is applied, especially in winter.

(4) When using moxibustion for the first time, pay attention to dosage. Start from a small dose and increase step by step. For example, use a small moxa cone, or apply it for a shorter time, or use less moxa cones, then gradually increase the dosage.

(5) Pay attention to when to use moxibustion, for example, apply it to patients with insomnia before sleep. Do not apply moxibustion before meals and immediately after meals.

(6) Be careful to observe patients during moxibustion to prevent moxibustion-sickness which leads to dizziness, blurry eyes, nausea, pale face, palpitation, sweating and etc. , and even faint in severe cases. Once happen, stop moxibustion immediately and let patients lie down and rest.

(7) Care should be taken to the temperature of moxibustion. For people with diabetes, limb numbness, dysesthesia or children, adjust a proper moxibustion temperature to prevent burning.

(8) Prevent infection. No treatment is needed if there are small blisters. For the large

one, break it and draw the fluid with a disposable syringe after disinfection with iodophor cotton balls, and then bandaged with a sterile gauze.

第三节 刮 痧
（*Guasha*）

刮痧是中医传统的自然疗法,以脏腑经络学说为理论基础,用器具(牛角、玉石、陶瓷片)等在皮肤相关部位刮拭,使局部皮肤发红充血,改善局部微循环,以达到疏通经络、活血化瘀的目的。刮痧可以扩张毛细血管,增加汗腺分泌,促进血液循环,使局部皮肤发红充血,改善局部的微循环,从而起到解毒祛邪、清热解表、行气止痛、强健心肺和增强机体自身免疫能力的效用。

刮痧疗法最早可追溯到旧石器时代,人们患病时往往会本能地用手或石片抚摩、捶击体表某一部位,逐渐发现疾病疼痛得到了缓解。通过长期的发展与积累,逐步形成了砭石治病的方法。砭石是针刺术、刮痧法的萌芽阶段,刮痧疗法可以说是砭石疗法的延续、发展或另一种存在形式。到了青铜器时代,人们发明了冶金技术,随着冶金技术的发展,可以冶炼出铁。铁比砭石更加精细,应用也更加广泛。随着针灸经络理论的发展,刮痧在民间开始流传,人们用边沿钝滑的铜钱、汤匙、瓷杯盖、钱币、玉器、纽扣等器具,在皮肤表面相关经络部位反复刮动,直到皮下出现红色或紫色瘀斑,来达到疏通腠理、祛邪外出、调理痧症的作用。在不断的实践中,被逐渐演绎成一种自然疗法。

一、刮痧原理（Principle of *Guasha*）

刮拭经络穴位,通过良性刺激,充分发挥营卫之气的作用,使经络穴位处充血,改善局部微循环,起到祛除邪气,疏通经络,舒筋理气,祛风散寒,清热除湿,活血化瘀,消肿止痛的功效,增强机体自身潜在的抗病能力和免疫功能,从而达到扶正祛邪、防病治病的作用。现代科学证明,刮痧可以扩张毛细血管,增加汗腺分泌,促进血液循环,对于高血压、中暑、肌肉酸痛等所致的风寒痹症都有立竿见影之效。

二、刮痧作用（Function of *Guasha*）

（一）疏通经络,调和气血

气血(通过经络系统)的传输对人体起着濡养、温煦等作用。刮痧使毛细血管扩张,促进血液循环,改善微循环。刮痧作用于肌表,使经络通畅,气血通达,则瘀血化散,凝滞固塞得以崩解消除,全身气血通达无碍,经络得以通畅,局部疼痛得以减轻或消失。

（二）调整阴阳，活络消炎

"阴平阳秘，精神乃治"。中医十分强调机体阴阳关系的平衡。刮痧对人体功能有双向调节作用，可以改善和调整脏腑功能，使脏腑阴阳得到平衡。刮痧能加强局部新陈代谢，刺激免疫功能，起到消炎的作用。

（三）活血祛瘀，排出毒素

刮痧可调节肌肉的收缩和舒张，使组织间压力得到调节，以促进刮拭组织周围的血液循环。增加组织流量，从而起到"活血化瘀""祛瘀生新"的作用。刮痧促进毛细血管扩张和血液循环，促进汗腺分泌、尿液排泄，使体内废物、毒素加速排出，最终清除沉淀在皮肤深处的毒素和代谢废物，达到排毒祛邪的功效。

三、刮痧器具（Tools for *Guasha*）

刮痧的器具主要是刮痧板，古时候人们刮痧所用的器具十分简单，主要是边缘比较圆滑的东西，如梳子、搪瓷杯盖等都可以用来刮痧。现在水牛角制品、玉制品较受人们欢迎。

（一）水牛角

水牛角，味辛、咸，性寒，辛可发散行气、活血消肿；咸能软坚润下；寒能清热解毒、凉血定惊。所以牛角刮痧板可以达到发散行气、清热解毒、活血化瘀的作用。且水牛角质地坚韧、光滑耐用、原料丰富、加工简便。注意忌热水长时间浸泡、火烤或电烤；刮痧后需立即把刮板擦干，涂上橄榄油，并存放于刮板套内。

（二）玉石

玉，味甘，性平，入肺经，润心肺，清肺热。玉石具有润肤生肌、清热解毒、镇静安神、辟邪散浊等作用。玉制刮痧板有助于行气活血、疏通经络，且其质地温润光滑，便于持握，因其触感舒适，适宜面部刮痧；注意用完后要注意清洁，避免碰撞，避免与化学试剂接触。

刮痧的介质，其实是刮痧所用润滑剂，可以增加皮肤与刮痧板间的润滑度，减少阻力，避免刮痧时损伤皮肤，同时具有药物外用治疗作用，可增强刮痧的疗效。常用刮痧介质是刮痧油，是用油性润滑介质添加具有活血化瘀、行气、解毒等功效的中药成分，制成刮痧油，具有清热解毒，活血化瘀，疏通经络，扩张毛细血管，消毒止痛，促进新陈代谢，促进血液循环，促使出痧的作用，除头部刮痧外，其他治疗部位的皮肤上，一般都应先涂抹刮痧油再进行刮痧。

四、刮痧手法（Technique of *Guasha*）

1. 刮板的握法　施术者用手掌握住刮板，治疗时刮板厚的一面对手掌，保健时刮板薄的一面对手掌。

2. 刮拭方向　顺着颈、背、腹、上肢、下肢这个顺序，从上向下刮拭，胸部从内向外刮拭。

3. 补刮、泻刮　通常来说，顺着经络的走行进行刮拭，即为补刮；逆着经络的走行进行刮拭即为泻刮。

4. 平补平泻法　即"平刮法"，有3种刮拭手法。第一种为按压力大，速度慢；第二种为按压力小，速度快；第三种为按压力中等，速度适中。具体应用时根据患者病情和体质而灵活选用。平补平泻法是介于补法与泻法之间的一种手法。

5. 刮痧时间　如果施术者用泻刮或平补平泻手法进行刮痧，每个部位一般要刮3～5分钟；用补刮手法时，每个部位的刮拭时间为5～10分钟。刮板与刮拭方向一般保持在45～90度进行刮痧。刮痧板一定要消毒。刮痧时间一般每个部位刮3～5分钟，最长不超20分钟。对于一些不出痧或出痧少的患者，不可强求出痧，以患者感到舒服为原则。刮痧次数一般是第一次刮完等3～5天，痧退后再进行第二次刮治。出痧后1～2天，皮肤可能轻度疼痛、发痒，这些反应属正常现象。保健刮痧则无严格的时间限制，以患者的感觉为原则，直到满意、舒服为止。

6. 刮痧力度　刮痧时用力要均匀，力度由轻到重，以患者能够承受为度，根据患者的体质选择不同的刮拭力量。其中，小儿、年老体弱患者以及面部刮痧用力宜轻，体质强健患者或脊柱两侧，下肢等肌肉较为丰满部位的刮痧用力偏重。

五、刮痧适应证（Indications of *Guasha*）

1. 内科病症　感受外邪引起的感冒发热、头痛、咳嗽、呕吐、腹泻以及高温中暑等，急性和慢性支气管炎、肺部感染、哮喘、心脑血管疾病、失眠、多梦、神经官能症等病症都适应刮痧治疗。

2. 外科病症　以疼痛为主要症状的各种外科病症（如急性扭伤），感受风、寒、湿邪导致的各种软组织疼痛，以及坐骨神经痛、肩周炎、落枕、慢性腰痛、风湿性关节炎、类风湿性关节炎、骨质增生、皮肤瘙痒症、荨麻疹、痤疮、湿疹、脱发等。

3. 儿科病症　营养不良、食欲不振、腹泻、生长发育迟缓、小儿感冒发热、遗尿等。

4. 五官科病症　牙痛、鼻炎、鼻窦炎、咽喉肿痛、视力减退、弱视、青少年假性近视、急性结膜炎、耳聋、耳鸣。

5. 妇科病症　痛经、闭经、月经不调、乳腺增生、乳腺炎、盆腔炎、产后病等。

6. 保健　病后康复、强身健体及减肥、美容等。

六、刮痧禁忌证（Contraindications of *Guasha*）

1. 患有严重心脑血管疾病、肝肾功能不全、心力衰竭等危重患者。因为刮痧会使人皮下充血,血液循环增快,从而增加心、肺、肝、肾的负担,加重病情。

2.妇女四期,即行经期、妊娠期、哺乳期、更年期应慎用。

3.如果体表出现疖肿、破溃、疮痈、斑疹、炎症等不明原因的包块时应禁止刮痧,否则将有可能会导致患处的感染与扩散。

4.凡体表处有溃烂、损伤、炎症等情况时,均不能用本疗法,初愈的患处也不可擅自采用。

5.急性扭伤部位、因创伤导致的疼痛部位及骨折部位应禁止刮痧,以防发生伤口出血。

6.如患有接触性皮肤病、传染病,应忌用刮痧,以防疾病传播。

7.有出血倾向的患者,如贫血、白血病、血小板减少症患者都应该禁止刮痧。

8.过度饥饱、过度疲劳及醉酒者禁忌大力和大面积刮痧,以防引起虚脱。

9.患者的心尖搏动处、眼睛、唇部、舌、耳、鼻、部位都是刮痧的禁止部位,以防充血。

七、刮痧注意事项(Precautions of *Guasha*)

1.进行刮痧治疗时,必须暴露皮肤,刮痧治疗时应注意室内保暖,尤其是在冬季应避免寒冷与风口。夏季刮痧时,应回避风扇直接吹刮拭部位。选择一个比较舒适的体位,以便于刮拭。

2.刮痧前,要把刮痧工具进行严格消毒,防止交叉感染。另外,还须认真检查刮痧器具,再涂抹刮痧油进行刮治,预防对皮肤造成的损伤。

3.前一次刮痧部位的痧斑未退之前,不宜在原处进行再次刮拭出痧。再次刮痧时间需间隔3~6天,以皮肤上痧退为标准。

4.刮痧前一定要与被施者解释清楚刮痧的一般常识,消除其恐惧心理,取得配合,以便于治疗的顺利进行。

5.施术者的双手应该进行全面消毒,被施者不应在过饥、过饱及过度紧张的情况下进行刮痧治疗。

6.施术者不可一味追求出痧,进而用重手法或延长刮痧时间,出痧的结果受多方面因素影响。一般情况下,血瘀之证出痧多;实证、热证出痧多;虚证、寒证出痧少;服药过多者,特别服用激素类药物不易出痧;肥胖者与肌肉丰满的人不易出痧;阴经较阳经不易出痧;室温低时不易出痧。所以,施术者用力一定要均匀、适中、由轻渐重,不要过于追求出痧。

7.如果被施术者是婴幼儿或者老年人,用力应以轻度为宜。

8.施术过程中,要不断询问被施者的感受。如遇到晕刮,如精神疲惫,头晕目眩、面色苍白、恶心欲吐,出冷汗、心慌、四肢发凉或血压下降、神志不清时应立即停止刮痧,并帮助患者缓解不适。

9. 刮痧疗法使汗孔开泄，邪气外排，要消耗体内部分的津液，故刮痧后需饮温水1 杯，最好是淡盐水，休息 20 ~ 25 分钟为宜。

10. 对于某些复杂危重的患者，除用刮痧治疗，更应配合其他诸如药物治疗，以免延误病情。

11. 刮痧出痧后 30 分钟以内忌洗凉水澡。

Guasha（scraping）is a conventional and natural therapy of TCM, guided by the theory of viscera and meridians. It uses special tools（such as ox horn, jade and ceramicv chip）to scrap on the skin, thereby making the skin flushed and congested, which can dredge meridians, improve blood circulation and remove blood stasis.

By dilating capillaries and increase sweating, it can also detoxify, dispel pathogenic factors, clear the heat, promote *qi* flow, and relieve pain. And it strengthens the function of heart and lung and enhances immunity.

The therapy can be traced back to the Paleolithic Age. When people got sick, they often instinctively touched and beat a certain part of the body with their hands or stone pieces, and gradually found that pain could be relieved.

Then *bian*-stone needling came into being through long-term development.

It can be said that acupuncture and *guasha* grew out of it.

In the Bronze Age, iron was created by metallurgical technology, which is finer than *bian*-stone. With the development of acupuncture meridian theory, *guasha* became widespread.

People used copper coins, spoons, porcelain cup covers, coins, jade, buttons with round and smooth edge to scrape repeatedly on the certain part of skin until red or purple spot under the skin appeared, so as to dredge interstice and striae, eliminate pathogenic factors and regulate *sha* disease.

Then it gradually became a natural therapy in practice.

1　Principle of *Guasha*

Scraping acupoints in meridian as benign stimulation brings about congestion, giving full play the role of the *qi* of *ying*-nutrients and *wei*-defence, which can dispel evil-*qi*, dredg meridians, relax muscles and regulate *qi*, remove wind and cold, clear away heat and dampness, promote blood circulation and remove blood stasis, reduce swelling and relieve pain. Its goal is to enhance immunity to prevent and treat diseases. Modern science has proved that scraping can dilate capillaries, increase sweat gland secretion and promote blood circulation, and has an immediate effect on wind-cold *bi*-impediment disease caused by hypertension, heatstroke and muscle soreness.

2　Function of *Guasha*

2.1　Dredging Meridians and Harmonizing *Qi* and Blood

Qi and blood (transported through meridian system) plays a role in nourishing and warming human body. Scraping dilates capillaries to improve local blood circulation. Scraping on the skin makes the meridians unobstructed and *qi* and blood flow smoothly, so that blood stasis can be removed and pain can be relieved.

2.2　Adjusting *Yin* and *Yang*, Activating Collaterals and Allay Inflammation

"Only when yin and yang are in balance can spirit be normal," which means TCM emphasizes the balance of *yin* and *yang*. Scraping can improve and adjust the functions of viscera, thus striking the balance between *yin* and *yang* of viscera. It can also strengthen local metabolism, stimulate immune function and allay inflammation.

2.3　Promoting Blood Circulation, Removing Blood Stasis and Toxins

Scraping can adjust the contraction and relaxation of muscles, regulate the pressure between tissues to promote the local blood circulation.

Increased blood flow helps to promote blood circulation and remove blood stasis.

Scraping promotes capillary dilatation, blood circulation and sweat gland secretion to accelerate the discharge of wastes and toxins, thus achieving the effect of detoxification and removal of pathogenic factors.

3　Tools for *Guasha*

People mainly use scraping plates as *guasha* tools. What ancient people used for scraping are simple, most of which have smooth edges, such as combs and enamel cup covers. Now buffalo horn and jade products are more popular.

3.1　Buffalo Horn

It is pungent and salty in taste, and cold in nature. The pungently can disperse and promote *qi* and blood circulation, and reduce swelling. The salty can soften hardness and moisten dryness. The cold can clear away heat and detoxify, cool blood and arrest convulsion. Therefore, *guasha* plate made of the horn has the same effect. And buffalo is hard, smooth, durable, available and easy to make. But do not soak it in hot water for a long time or heat it with fire or electricity. After scraping, clean and dry the scraper immediately, coat it with olive oil, and store it in the scraper cover.

3.2　Jade

Jade, sweet in taste and neutral in nature, enters lung meridian, so it can moisten heart and lung, and clear lung heat.

It also has the function of moistening skin, promoting granulation, clearing away heat and detoxifying, calming mind, eliminating pathogenic factors and dispelling turbidity. The scraping plate made of jade is helpful to promote *qi* and blood circulation, dredge meridians.

As it is smooth and easy to hold, it is suitable for facial scraping.

Clean it after use, and avoid collision and contact with chemical reagents.

The medium of *guasha* is actually the lubricant used for scraping, which can increase the lubrication between skin and scraping plate lest skin be injured. Meanwhile, its medical effect can enhance the curative effect of *guasha*.

The commonly used medium is *guasha* oil, which is made of Chinese medicine with the effects of promoting blood circulation and removing blood stasis, promoting *qi* circulation and detoxifying. The oil should be applied before scraping to the skin except for the head.

4　Technique of *Guasha*

4.1　Grasping

Practitioners should hold the scraper in the hand, with the thick side facing the palm during treatment and the thin side facing the palm during health care.

4.2　Direction

Scrape from top to bottom along neck, back, abdomen, upper limbs and lower limbs, but scrape the chest from center to periphery.

4.3　Scraping as reinforcing and reducing

Generally speaking, scraping as reinforcing refers to scrape in the same direction as meridians and the latter refers to scrape in reverse direction.

4.4　Scraping as balanced reinforcing and reducing

It is another scraping technique, which is also called balanced scraping, and has three categories. The first is to scrape slowly with high pressure; the second is to scrape fast with low pressure and the third is to scrape at moderate speed and with moderate pressure. Choose the proper one according to the patient's condition. The method is a technique between the mentioned above.

4.5　Duration

It takes 3–5 minutes to scrape each part with reducing technique and balanced one, and

5 – 10 minutes with reinforcing one.

Hold the tool at a 45° – 90° angle. Scraping plates must be disinfected. Do not scrape for more than 20 minutes each part. Do not scrape for the occurrence of *sha*. Try the best to let patients feel comfortable.

Carry the second scraping 3 – 5 days after the first one (when *sha* disappears). Normally, patients may feel slightly painful and itchy 1–2 days after scraping, which is normal. There is no strict time limit of scraping for health care, and try the best to make patients satisfied and comfortable.

4.6　Intensity

Apply even and mild pressure, and gradually increase intensity to determine how much force the patients can handle. Apply a proper intensity according to the patient's physique.

Scrape with light pressure for children, the elderly, the infirm, and on facial region, while scrape with heavy pressure for those who are strong, or on muscular parts such as both sides of spine and lower limbs.

5　Indications of *Guasha*

5.1　Medical Diseases

Cold, fever, headache, cough, vomiting, diarrhea and heat stroke caused by exogenous pathogens, acute or chronic bronchitis, lung infection, asthma, cardiovascular and cerebrovascular diseases, insomnia, dreaminess and neurosis.

5.2　Surgical Diseases

Various surgical diseases with pain as the main symptom (such as acute sprain), soft tissue pain caused by wind, cold and dampness, sciatica, scapulohumeral periarthritis, stiff neck, chronic low back pain, rheumatic and rheumatoid arthritis, hyperosteogeny, skin pruritus, urticaria, acne, eczema, hair loss, etc.

5.3　Pediatric Diseases

Malnutrition, loss of appetite, diarrhea, growth retardation, children's cold and fever, enuresis, etc.

5.4　ENT Diseases

Toothache, rhinitis, sinusitis, sore throat, poor eyesight, amblyopia, juvenile pseudomyopia, acute conjunctivitis, deafness and tinnitus.

5.5　Gynecological Diseases

Dysmenorrhea, amenorrhea, irregular menstruation, hyperplasia of mammary glands, mastitis, pelvic inflammatory disease and postpartum diseases.

5.6　Health Care

Rehabilitation, physical fitness, weight loss, beauty, etc.

6　Contraindications of *Guasha*

（1）It is not allowed to apply *guasha* to patients with severe cardiovascular and cerebro-vascular diseases, liver and kidney insufficiency, heart failure. Because it will aggravate the disease by increasing the burden on heart, lung, liver and kidney due to congestion and accelerated blood circulation.

（2）It should be used with caution to women in menstruation, pregnancy, lactation and menopause.

（3）It is forbidden to use *guasha* if there are furuncle, ulceration, sores, macula and inflammation on skin, otherwise it may lead to infection and spread.

（4）It is forbidden to scrape on the skin with ulceration, injury, inflammation. The newly recovered part cannot be scraped either.

（5）To prevent wound bleeding, it is forbidden to use *guasha* on areas of acute sprain, pain area caused by trauma and fracture.

（6）To prevent the spread of diseases, it is forbidden to apply *guasha* to people with contact dermatosis and infectious diseases

（7）It is prohibited to apply *guasha* to people with hemorrhagic disease, such as anemia, leukemia and thrombocytopenia.

（8）To prevent collapse, it is forbidden to apply *guasha* to people who are famished, over-tired and drunk.

（9）To prevent congestion, it is forbidden to scrape on apex beat position, eyes, lips, tongue, ears and nose.

7　Precautions of *Guasha*

（1）On performing *guasha*, expose the treatment parts and keep warm, avoid wind and cold especially in winter. When scraping in summer, the treatment parts should not be blown directly by the fan. Let patients choose a comfortable position for scraping.

（2）Before scraping, disinfect scraping tools to prevent cross infection. In addition, it is necessary to carefully check the scraping tools, and then apply scraping oil to prevent skin being injured.

（3）It is not advisable to scrape again before the *sha* disappears. The interval of scraping should be 3–6 days, and it depends on when *sha* disappears.

(4) Before scraping, explain the general knowledge of scraping clearly to the patients to get rid of their fear and for their cooperation, so as to facilitate the process.

(5) Hands disinfection is necessary. Do not perform *guasha* when patients are famished, overeating and highly anxious.

(6) Do not apply heavy pressure or prolong the duration in order to scrape for the occurance of *sha* because whether *sha* occurs depends on many factors. Generally, there is more *sha* if patients suffer from blood stasis syndrome or excess and heat syndromes; and less *sha* if deficiency and cold syndrome. *Sha* will not easily come out for those who take too much medicine, especially hormone drugs, and who are obese or muscular. Also, *sha* appears more when scraping on *yang* meridians than *yin* meridians. Besides, there will be less *sha* when room temperature is low. Therefore, be careful to apply suitable pressure in proper way.

(7) For infant or the elderly, apply mild force.

(8) Keep asking the patients feelings when scraping.

In case of *guasha* – sickness manifested as mental exhaustion, dizziness, pale face, nausea, vomiting, cold sweat, palpitation, cold limbs, decreased blood pressure and unconsciousness, stop scraping immediately and help the patient relieve discomfort.

(9) *Guasha* can open pores to discharge evil *qi*, which will consume body fluids. Therefore, it is advisable to drink a cup of lukewarm water (salt water is better) after *guasha* and rest for 20–25 minutes.

(10) Patients with some diseases should also have medical treatment, in addition to *guasha*.

(11) Avoid taking a cold bath within 30 minutes after scraping.

第四节 拔 罐
（Cupping）

一、拔罐原理（Principle of Cupping）

（一）刺激作用

拔罐疗法通过排气造成罐内负压，使罐得以紧紧附着于皮肤表面，牵拉了神经、肌肉、血管以及皮下的腺体，可引起一系列神经内分泌反应，调节血管舒缩功能和血管的通透性从而改善局部血液循环。这种吸拔力可以通过皮肤感受器和血管感受器对大脑皮质产生刺激作用,使之兴奋或抑制。

（二）负压效应

拔罐的负压作用使局部迅速充血、瘀血,小毛细血管破裂,红细胞被破坏,发生溶血现象。红细胞中血红蛋白的释放对机体是一种良性刺激,它可通过神经系统对组织器官的功能进行双向调节,同时促进白细胞的吞噬作用,提高皮肤对外界变化的敏感性及耐受力,从而增强机体的免疫力。其次,负压的强大吸拔力可使汗毛孔充分张开,汗腺和皮脂腺的功能受到刺激而加强,皮肤表层衰老细胞脱落,从而使体内的毒素、废物得以加速排出。

（三）温热作用

拔罐局部的温热作用使血管扩张、血流量增加,促进局部血液循环,加强新陈代谢,增强血管壁的通透性和细胞的吞噬能力。拔罐处血管紧张度及黏膜渗透性改变,淋巴循环加速,吞噬作用加强,增强机体抵抗力,另外,溶血现象的慢性刺激对人体起到了保健功能。

二、拔罐作用(Function of Cupping)

（一）疏通经络

人体的经络承担着人体的气血运行、输布、濡养、联络、调节作用。拔罐的治病作用,是在相应的穴位或部位上,通过罐的负压作用,疏通被阻的经络通道,进而激发经络之气,使其发挥特有的生理作用,从而达到调节机体平衡的作用。

（二）调理气血

人体的脏腑器官凭借气血的濡养,保持着正常发育生长,发挥着各自生理功能。如因某种因素气血发生障碍时,则出现气血偏盛、偏衰的不同证候。拔罐则可在相应的穴位或部位上,使之充血或出血,从而疏通了瘀滞,补益了不足而趋于平衡,在脏腑、经络气血凝滞或脉络空虚时,引导经络之气往来输布,鼓动经脉气血,濡养脏腑、组织,鼓舞正气,加强机体祛除病邪能力,从而使疾病得以祛除。

（三）祛邪扶正

如果机体内外发生湿热邪毒疖肿的情况时,可以通过拔火罐使相应部位瘀阻消散,托毒排脓,改善充血或出血,拔出毒血,调补正气,使之湿热以清,邪毒以解,疖肿以消,扶正祛邪。

（四）活血止痛

拔罐疗法通过对腧穴局部的负压吸附作用,使体表组织产生充血、瘀血等变化,改善血液循环,使经络气血通畅,瘀血化散。对局部组织来说,可以消肿止痛。

三、拔罐常用工具（Common Tools for Cupping）

（一）玻璃罐

火罐法的首选工具。

优点：罐口平滑、不易损伤皮肤，质地透明，可以直接观察罐内瘀血、充血情况，便于掌握拔罐的治疗程度。

缺点：易破碎。

（二）陶罐

陶罐由陶土烧制而成。

优点：吸附力大，治疗效果好。

缺点：质地较重、容易破碎。

（三）竹罐

竹罐由竹竿打磨制成，水罐法的首选工具。

优点：价格低廉、取材方便、轻巧易制、不易破碎。

缺点：吸力小、容易爆裂漏气。

（四）抽气罐

抽气罐由化学材料和吸防气装置加工组成。

优点：容易操作、便于抽气、可避免烫伤。

缺点：无温热效应、疗效相对较差。

四、常用拔罐方法（Common Cupping Methods）

（一）拔罐

拔罐是最简单基本的方法。一只手持罐，另一只手拿已点着火的探子，将着火的探子在罐中晃上几晃后，撤出，将罐迅速放在要治疗的部位，然后用手轻轻拔一拔罐子，看是否吸上了。拔罐时应注意：不要将探子上的乙醇抹在罐子口上，也不要将探子上的乙醇滴落在患者的皮肤上，否则有可能会烫伤患者。

（二）闪罐

将已拔上的罐子迅速取下，然后再反复操作吸拔多次，直至皮肤出现潮红为止。闪罐法多用于虚寒证，或肌肉萎缩，或需重点刺激的穴位。闪罐时应注意：闪罐时罐子本身的温度较高，应备多个罐子，交替使用，以防烫伤患者的皮肤。

（三）走罐

在罐口或欲拔罐部位涂一些凡士林油膏等润滑剂，再将罐拔住，在罐子拔上以后，用一只手或两只手抓住罐子,微微上提,推拉罐体在患者的皮肤上移动,用右手握住罐子,向上、下、左、右需要拔罐的部位往返推动,至所拔部位的皮肤潮红、充血甚或瘀血时,将罐起下。

（四）留针拔罐

此法是将针刺和拔罐相结合应用的一种方法。先在治疗部位或穴位上进行针刺,即先针刺待得气后留针,再以针为中心点将火罐拔上,留置 10～15 分钟,然后起罐拔针。

（五）刺血拔罐

此法又称刺络拔罐。即在应拔部位的皮肤消毒后,用三棱针点刺出血或用皮肤针叩打后再行拔罐,使之出血,以加强刺血治疗的作用。一般针后拔罐留置 10～15 分钟。

五、拔罐适应证（Indications of Cupping）

（一）内科疾病

感冒、咳嗽、哮喘、心悸、失眠、健忘、呕吐、反胃、腹泻、便秘、腹痛、胃下垂等病症。

（二）外科疾病

急性阑尾炎、乳腺炎、急性胆绞痛、急性胰腺炎、急性输尿管结石、疖肿、毒蛇咬伤等病症。

（三）骨科疾病

落枕、颈椎病、肘关节痛、膝关节痛、髋部病变、腰椎间盘突出症、腰肌劳损、急性腰扭伤、肩关节周围炎、类风湿性骨关节炎等病症。

（四）妇科疾病

月经过少、经闭、痛经、月经不调、盆腔炎等病症。

（五）儿科疾病

百日咳、哮喘、消化不良、遗尿、小儿疳积、小儿呕吐、泄泻、腮腺炎等病症。

（六）皮肤科疾病

带状疱疹、皮肤瘙痒、荨麻疹、痤疮等疾病。

六、拔罐禁忌证（Contraindications of Cupping）

1. 皮肤局部破溃或高度过敏,以及患皮肤传染病的患者不宜拔罐。过饥、过饱、醉酒、过度劳累等不宜拔罐。

2. 形体消瘦,皮肤失去了弹性而松弛者及毛发多的部位不宜拔罐。急性骨关节炎、急性软组织损伤,局部忌用拔罐疗法。

3. 重症、病情严重、心肺功能不全、心力衰竭、呼吸衰竭、肾衰者不宜拔罐。

4. 妊娠期妇女的下腹部、腰骶部及合谷、三阴交等穴不宜拔罐。

5. 有出血倾向疾病,如血友病、血小板减少、紫癜、白血病等患者,不宜使用拔罐法。

6. 颈部及其他体表大血管处、眼、耳、乳头、前后阴、静脉曲张、癌肿、外伤者不宜拔罐。

7. 精神分裂症、抽搐、高度神经质及不合作者不宜拔罐。

七、拔罐注意事项(Precautions of Cupping)

1. 拔罐时要选择适当的体位和肌肉丰满的部位。若体位不当或有所移动及骨骼凸凹不平、毛发较多的部位,均不可用。

2. 应该根据个体差异确定留罐时间,一般成人为 10～15 分钟,儿童酌减。

3. 拔罐前仔细检查罐口周围是否光滑,有无破损,以免损伤患者皮肤。

4. 拔罐时要根据所拔部位的面积大小而选择大小适宜的罐。患者在初次治疗时,应先选用小拔罐,轻刺激,动作必须迅速,才能使罐拔紧,吸附有力。

5. 操作过程中应注意观察患者的反应,如有不适应立即起罐,过程中注意保暖。

6. 用火罐时应注意避免灼伤或烫伤皮肤。起罐后皮肤上的深红色斑为正常现象,告知患者数日可消退,不必担心。若烫伤或留罐时间太长而皮肤起水疱时,小的无须处理,可自行吸收,仅敷以消毒纱布,防止擦破即可。水疱较大时,用消毒针将水疱刺破放出水液,涂以龙胆紫药水或用消毒纱布包敷,以防感染。

7. 拔罐后多饮温开水,3 日内禁止洗澡,洗澡时拔罐部位不能用力摩擦,有水疱者可根据情况延长禁止洗澡时间,必要时每日或隔日清洁换药一次直至痊愈。

8. 儿童拔罐时间不宜过长,力度不宜过大,留罐时间不宜过长。

9. 皮肤有过敏、溃疡、水肿者,及大血管分布部位,不宜拔罐。高热抽搐者,以及孕妇的腹部、腰骶部,亦不宜拔罐。

1 Principle of Cupping

1.1 Stimulation

With this method, negative pressure is created inside the cup to consum the air thereby making the cup suck itself onto the skin. It will cause a series of neuroendocrine reactions by pulling nerves, muscles, blood vessels and subcutaneous glands, which can regulate vasomotor function and vascular permeability, thus improving local blood circulation.

This suction force can stimulate the cerebral cortex through skin and vascular receptors by exciting or inhibiting it.

1.2 Negative Pressure

Local congestion and blood stasis will occur because of the rupture of small capillaries and red blood cells (also called hemolysis) caused by negative pressure.

As the red blood cell ruptures, it will release hemoglobin, which is a benign stimulus to the body. It can regulate the functions of tissues and organs through the nervous system, promote the phagocytosis of white blood cells, decrease the susceptibility and improve the endruance capability of skin to external changes, thus enhancing immunity.

Besides, the strong suction force caused by negative pressure can fully open pores, strengthen the functions of stimulated sweat glands and sebaceous glands and help senescent cells on the skin fall off, thus accelerating the discharge of toxins and wastes.

1.3 Warming

Blood vessels will be dilated by the warming effect, in which blood flow increases. It can promote local blood circulation, strengthen metabolism, and enhances the permeability of blood vessel and phagocytosis of cells.

The immunity of body can also be enhanced by accelerated lymphatic circulation and strengthened phagocytosis due to the changes of vascular tension and mucosal permeability. In addition, chronic stimulation of hemolysis plays an active role in health protection.

2 Function of Cupping

2.1 Dredging Meridian

The meridian of human body is the passage where qi and blood circulate, distribute, nourish, interconnect and regulate.

Adopting cupping therapy can dredge the unobstructed meridian through the negative pressure on the certain acupoints or parts, and then stimulate the qi of meridian, so that it can function as normal, thus maintaining the balance of the body.

2.2 Regulating *Qi* and Blood

Thanks to the nourishment of qi and blood, the viscera and organs of human body develop and function normally.

When qi and blood are blocked for some reason, there will be different syndromes of excessive or deficient qi and blood.

The congestion or bleeding caused by cupping on certain acupoints or parts can remove blood stasis. In this way, meridian qi can be distributed and transported without obstruction. Qi and blood continue to nourish viscera and tissues, and healthy qi are strengthened to dispel pathogenic factors, which helps to prevent and treat diseases.

2.3 Eliminating Pathogenic factors and Strengthening Healthy *Qi*

Fire cupping can be used to treat furuncle due to damp−heat by dissipating the stasis, detoxifying and expelling pus, and promoting congestion or bleeding to remove the toxin. In this way, healthy *qi* can be consolidated. Therefore, it helps to clear damp heat, expelling pathogenic toxin, get rid of furuncle and reinforce healthy *qi*.

2.4 Promoting Blood Circulation and Relieving Pain

The congestion and blood stasis caused by cupping through negative pressure on acupoints can improve blood circulation, smooth the flow of *qi* and blood in meridians.

It has the effect of reducing swelling and relieving pain on local tissue.

3 Common Tools for Cupping

3.1 Glass Cup

It is the preferred tool for fire cupping method.

Advantages: The rim of glass cup is smooth, so it is not easy to damage skin. Since it is transparent, the congestion and blood stasis at the site can be directly observed so as to control the treatment.

Disadvantages: Fragile.

3.2 Pottery Cup

It is made of clay.

Advantages: Have great adsorption force and desirable treatment effect.

Disadvantages: Heavy and fragile.

3.3 Bamboo Cup

It is made of polished bamboo and the preferred tool for water-suction method.

Advantages: Low-cost, available, light, easy to make and sturdy.

Disadvantages: Little absorptive force, easy to leak air.

3.4 Suction Cup

It is composed of chemical materials and air suction and leakage prevention devices.

Advantages: Easy to manipulate, easy to withdraw air and avoid scalding.

Disadvantages: No warming effect and relatively poor therapeutic effect.

4 Common Cupping Methods

4.1 Cupping

It is the simplest and most basic method. Put the ignited paper or an alcohol cotton ball into the cup and take it out immediately.

Then place the cup on the selected position. Gently pull out the cup by hand to see whether it is sucked in place.

Precautions:Do not leave the ethanol of the ignited object on the cup mouth and the patient's skin,otherwise it may scorch the skin.

4.2　Flash Cupping

Make the cup sucked on the skin and immediately remove it. Repeat the cause for several times until the skin becomes flush.

This method is extensively used to treat cold syndrome of deficiency type and amyotrophy,or stimulate acupoints.

Precautions:In this method,the cups are at high temperature,so prepare more cups for alternative use to prevent scalding the skin.

4.3　Sliding Cupping

Apply lubricants such as Vaseline to the cup mouth or the selected area of skin,the cup then is sucked to the skin. Hold the cup with one hand or two hands,then lift it slightly and slide it around and back to the selected area until the skin becomes flushed,congested or even bruised. Remove the cup.

4.4　Needle-retention Cupping

This method serves as therapy of both acupuncture and cupping. Insert the needle into a selected area or acupoint to induce needling sensation and retain the needle there.

Then place the cup with the fire twinkling method over the skin where the needle is retained,the needle being the center inside the cup. After 10-15 minutes,remove the cup and the needle.

4.5　Blood-letting and Cupping

This is also referred to as cupping with collateral-pricking.

After disinfecting the skin of the selected part,it is punctured with three-edged needle to cause bleeding, or tapped with cutaneous needle, then apply cupping to induce more bleeding,which enhances the treatment effect.

Generally,retain the cup for 10-15 minutes after acupuncture.

5　Indications of Cupping

5.1　Medical Diseases

Cold,cough,asthma,palpitation,insomnia,forgetfulness,vomiting,nausea,diarrhea,constipation,abdominal pain,gastroptosis,etc. and other diseases.

5.2 Surgical Diseases

Acute appendicitis, mastitis, acute biliary colic, acute pancreatitis, acute ureteral calculi, furuncle, venomous snake bite, etc.

5.3 Orthopedic Diseases

Stiff neck, cervical spondylosis, elbow arthritis, knee arthritis, hip diseases, lumbar disc herniation, lumbar muscle strain, acute lumbar sprain, scapulohumeral periarthritis, rheumatoid osteoarthritis, etc.

5.4 Gynecological Diseases

Hypomenorrhea, amenorrhea, dysmenorrhea, irregular menstruation, pelvic inflammation, etc.

5.5 Pediatric Diseases

Pertussis, asthma, indigestion, enuresis, infantile malnutrition, infantile vomiting, diarrhea, mumps, etc.

5.6 Dermatological Diseases

Herpes zoster, itchy skin, urticaria, acne, etc.

6 Contraindications of Cupping

(1) It is not advised to apply cupping to people with local skin ulcer, allergic skin or skin infection and people who are famished, overeating, drunk or overtired.

(2) It is not advised to apply cupping to those who are emaciated and who have less skin elasticity. And cupping is not effective on areas where there is excessive body hair. It is forbidden to apply cupping to people with acute osteoarthritis and acute soft tissue injury.

(3) It is not advised to apply cupping to people with serious illness, cardiopulmonary insufficiency, heart failure, respiratory failure and renal failure.

(4) It is not advised to apply cupping on areas like abdominal and sacral region of pregnant women as well as Hegu (LI4), Sanyinjiao (SP6) and other acupoints.

(5) It is not advised to apply cupping to people with hemorrhagic diseases, such as hemophilia, thrombocytopenia, purpura, leukemia, etc.

(6) It is not advised to apply cupping on neck, areas overlying large blood vessels, eyes, ears, nipples, urethra, genitalia and anus. People with varicose veins, cancer and trauma should not use either.

(7) It is forbidden to use cupping when patients suffer from schizophrenia, convulsions, hyperneuroticism and do not cooperate.

7　Precautions of Cupping

(1) The patients should select a comfortable position and muscular areas should be selected for treatment. Stop cupping if the position is improper or changes. Do not put on hairy or bony region.

(2) The time of retaining cups should be determined according to individual situation. Generally, leave the cups on adults for 10–15 minutes and on children for reasonably reduced time.

(3) It is necessary to check whether the cup mouth is smooth and unbroken before cupping, otherwise the skin may be injured.

(4) Cups in different sizes are used according to the cupping location. When patients first try cupping therapy, choose small cups and cup them to the skin rapidly so that the cups can be attached to the skin firmly.

(5) Attention should be paid to observe the patient's reaction during manipulation. Remove the cup immediately once patients feel uncomfortable. Keep warm during the operation.

(6) Avoid burning or scalding the skin when adopting fire cupping method.

It is normal that there may be crimson spot on the skin after cupping, and do not worry about that because it will disappear of its own accord.

However, if there are blisters caused by scalding or prolonged duration, the small one can be absorbed by itself so no treatment is needed. Only apply sterilized gauze to it to prevent rubbing.

But the large one should be treated by piercing with a sterilized needle to let the fluid flow out, then apply gentian violet or cover it with sterilized gauze to prevent infection.

(7) Drink more lukewarm water after cupping, and no bathing is allowed within three days. When taking a bath, the cupping site should not be rubbed hard. For patients with blisters, extend bathing – forbidden days according to circumstances. If necessary, clean and change fresh dressing for the wound once a day or every other day until recovery.

(8) For children, retain the cup for a shorter time and do not cup with strong pull.

(9) It is inadvisable to apply cupping to patients with skin allergy, ulcer and edema, and areas overlying large blood vessels.

第五节 中医保健操——八段锦
（Health Exercises of Traditional Chinese Medicine—*Baduan Jin*）

中医养生保健操通过舒缓的运动方式配合宁静的呼吸,进行养心安神的调节,从而疏通经络,改善脏腑功能,调畅精神,达到强身健体,祛病延年的目的。常见的保健操有八段锦、五禽戏、太极拳、易筋经等。在我国古老的导引术中,八段锦是流传最广,对导引术发展影响最大的一种。八段锦功法以脏腑为纲,具有调整脏腑功能的功效。

一、动作要领（Key Points）

1. 双手托天理三焦　自然站立,双足分开,两脚平行,与肩同宽。含胸收腹、平头正视,全身放松。两臂徐徐分别自左右身侧向上高举过头,十指交叉,翻转掌心极力向上托,使两臂充分伸展,同时缓缓抬头上看,目视两掌,眼睛跟随手的方向,此时缓缓吸气。翻转掌心朝下,在身前正落至胸高时,随落随翻转掌心再朝上,微低头,眼随手运。同进配以缓缓呼气。足跟亦随双手的托举而起落,如此两掌上托下落,练习4~8次。

2. 左右开弓似射雕　自然站立,重心右移,右腿微屈,左脚向左迈开一步,略比肩宽,两脚平行站立。身体下蹲成骑马步,双手虚握于两髋之外侧,随后自胸前向上划弧提至与乳平高处。手握拳,示指与拇指呈"八字形"撑开,左手缓缓向左平推,左臂展直,同时右臂屈肘向右拉回,右拳停于右肋前,拳心朝上,如拉弓状。视线通过左手示指凝视远方,意如弓箭在手,等机而射,稍作停顿后,拉伸1~2秒。随后转头向左,随即将身体上起,顺势将两手向下划弧收回胸前,并同时收回左腿,还原成自然站立。此为左式,右式反方向动作,右脚开步,搭手向上,右手在外,两手拉弓,重心左移,并脚。左右调换练习4~8次。最后一个动作结束,身体重心左移,右脚回收成开步站立,与肩同宽,膝关节微屈。回到预备式。

3. 调理脾胃须单举　自然站立,左手自身前成竖掌缓缓向上高举至头,然后翻转掌心向上,指尖向右,同时右掌心向下按,指尖朝前。左手向左外方托举,右手向下按,之后换右手掌上托,左手掌下按,重复上述动作。如此左右互换4~8次,最后左手俯掌在身前下落,同时引气血下行,全身随之放松,恢复自然站立。

4. 五劳七伤往后瞧　两脚自然平行站立,与肩同宽。两臂、双手自然下垂,气沉丹田。头颈带动脊柱缓缓向左拧转,两眼目视左后方,稍稍停顿,同时配合吸气,然后缓缓转正,头颈带动脊柱徐徐向右转,恢复前平视。同时配合呼气,全身放松。重复上述动作,头改为看向右后方,其余动作与上相同,如此左右后瞧各4~8次。最后一个动作结束,身体重心缓缓下降,膝关节微微弯曲,膝盖不可超过脚尖,两掌捧于腹前,掌心向上,目视前方。回到预备式。

5. 摇头摆尾去心火　两脚开,双膝下蹲,马步站立,上体稍向前探,两目平视,双手按在膝盖上,双肘外撑。以腰为轴,背部保持挺直,将躯干划弧摇转至左前方,左臂弯曲,右臂绷直,肘臂外撑,头与左膝呈一垂线,臀部向右下方撑劲,目视右足尖;稍停顿后,随即向相反方向,上身从左向右移动,重心缓缓移动到右脚,左腿微微拉伸,不可完全伸直。移动过程中,眼睛始终看着左脚面,保持含胸收腹、背部挺直。重复上述动作,方向从左边换为右边,动作交替进行各做 4～8 次。做完最后一个动作,身体重心右移,左脚回收成开步站立,与肩同宽;同时,两掌向外,掌心朝上,经两侧上举,到头顶上方,掌心相对,目视前方。

6. 双手攀足固肾腰　两脚平行站立,与肩同宽,两掌分按脐旁。两手向两侧分开,两臂伸直向上举起,同时两腿缓缓挺膝伸直,两手掌举过头顶,掌心向前,目视前方。稍停顿,两腿绷直,以腰为轴,身体前俯,两掌沿膀胱经向下滑动,上体向前俯身,两掌接着向下,顺着腿部到脚后跟,然后向前滑动到脚面,稍微停顿,随后沿脚外侧按摩至脚内侧。上体展直,同时两手沿两大腿内侧按摩至脐两旁。如此反复 4～8 次。最后一个动作结束,身体重心缓缓下降,膝关节微屈,两臂向前落于髋旁边,掌心向下,指尖向前,目视前方。

7. 攒拳怒目增气力　两脚开立,成马步桩,两手握拳分置腰间,双手握拳,拳眼向下。左拳向左前方缓缓击出,成立拳或俯拳,顺势头稍向左转。两眼通过左拳凝视远方,右拳同时后拉。然后左拳曲肘回收至腰侧,眼睛放松,拳眼向上,目视前方。如此左右交替各击出 4～8 次。最后身体重心右移,左脚回收,两腿并拢,成并步站立,两拳变掌,自然下垂于身体两侧,目视前方。

8. 背后七颠百病消　双腿并拢自然站立,双手自然下垂于身体两侧,目视前方。两脚跟提起,挺直腰背,提肛收腹,稍作停顿,将两脚跟下落着地。如此起落 4～8 次,并配合呼气,全身放松。

最后全身放松,自然呼吸,气沉丹田,稍微静息片刻。

二、练习要领（Practice Tips）

1. 松静自然,准确灵活　松是指精神与形体两方面的放松。自然指形体、呼吸、意念要自然协调。准确主要是指练功时的姿势与方法要正确,合乎规格。灵活,是指习练时对动作幅度的大小、姿势的高低、用力的大小、练习的数量、意念的运用、呼吸的调整等,都要根据自身情况灵活掌握。

2. 练养相兼,循序渐进　练是指形体运动、呼吸调整与心理调节有机结合的锻炼过程。养是通过上述练习,身体出现的轻松舒适、呼吸柔和、意守绵绵的静养状态。最开始练习要打好基础,慢慢达到姿势端庄,动作舒展,气势饱满,精神顶,动作形成自动化,从由外导内,慢慢转化为由内导外。

Practicing health exercises of TCM can nourish the heart and calm the mind through soothing exercise and quiet breathing, so as to dredge collaterals, improve viscera functions, regulate the spirit. In this way, one can build the body, cure diseases and prolong life.

Common health exercises include *Baduan Jin*, *Wuqin Xi*, *Taiji*, *Yijin Jing* and so on.

Among the ancient physical and breathing exercises in China, *Baduan Jin* is the most widespread and has the greatest influence on the development of the exercises.

Baduan Jin has the effect of adjusting viscera function.

1 Key Points

1.1 Holding the Hands High with Palms Up to Regulate *Sanjiao*

Stand with feet shoulder-width apart. Have chest and low abdomen slightly adducted. Look straight ahead and keep the whole body relaxed. Raise hands above the head from both sides of the body. Then interlace fingers with palms facing upward and fully stretch arms as if lifting an object. The eyes should follow the hands over the head. Inhale slowly at the same time. Rotate the palms downward. Exhale and lower the arms in front and push palms upward once hands are in front of the chest. Bow your head slightly with eyes following the hands. Raise heels off the ground in the movement of lifting arms. Repeat the routine 4-8 times.

1.2 Posing as an Archer Shooting Both Left-and Right-handed

Standing naturally. Shift the weight rightward with the right knee bent slightly, then step out the left foot (slightly wider than shoulders). Squat down in a horse-riding stance with feet standing in parallel. Move the crossed hands in front of the chest in anarc line. Hold hands in fist with index finger separated from thumb. Push left arm slowly to the left and extend it. Then pull the right elbow to the right until the right fist reaches in front of the right ribs. The posture is like pulling a bow. Look into distance following the tip of your left index finger. It seems as if you were pulling a bow to shoot. Stretch for 1-2 seconds. Then turn back the head, draw hands downward in an arc line and back to chest area. Stand up and move left leg back to return a natural standing. Do the same routine to the right. Start with your right leg to the right.

Raise crossed hands with right hand under left hand.

Do the bow-pulling gesture.

Then shift gravity center to the left and stand with feet together.

Repeat the whole process for 4-8 times.

When you finish the last routine, stand up and shift the weight leftward, then move your right leg back so the feet are parallel and shoulder-width apart.

Knees are bent slightly.

Return to the preparatory posture.

1.3 Holding One Arm Aloft to Regulate the Functions of the Spleen and Stomach

Stand naturally. Raise the left hand over the head and push upward with fingertips toward the right, and at the same time the right hand moves downward with the palm facing down and fingertips pointing forward.

Then change your hands and repeat the same process for 4-8 times.

Finally, lower the raising hand in front of the body and meanwhile, qi and blood are drawn down. Relax the whole body and stand naturally.

1.4 Looking Backwards to Prevent Sickness and Strain

The feet are parallel and at shoulder's width apart. Place both hands naturally alongside the body. Sink qi down to Dantian. Inhaling while slowly turning the head to the right side as far as possible, look back as much as possible. After a while, exhale and slowly return to the original position looking straight ahead. Relax the whole body. Do the same routine to the right and repeat the above actions for 4-8 times. When you finish the last routine, shift the weight downward. Bend the knees slightly, but do not exceed beyond the toes. Place the palms facing upward in front of the abdomen and look straight ahead. Return to the preparatory posture.

1.5 Swinging the Head and Lowering the Body to Eliminate the Heart fire.
Squat down in a Horse-riding stance with feet apart

Look straight ahead. Lean the torso and head forward. Put your hands on the knees with elbows outward. Take the waist as the axis. Keep the back straight. Swing the body to the left and forward with left arm bent and right arm extended. The head and left knee should be placed in a vertical line. Swing the buttocks to the right and look at the right toes. Hold the posture for a few seconds. Then move the upper body from left to right. The center of gravity slowly moves to the right foot and the left leg is slightly stretched. During the movement, always look at the left foot, and keep the back straight with chest and abdomen slightly adducted with the back. Do the same routine to the right and repeat the above actions for 4-8 times. When you finish the last routine, stand up and shift the weight rightward, then move your left leg back and keep the feet apart about shoulder-width. At the same time, raise hands over the top of head alongside body with palms facing upward, lift up on both sides. Palms face each other when reaching the top and look ahead.

1.6 Moving the Hands down the Back and Legs, and Touching the Feet to Strengthen the Kidneys and Waist

Keep feet in parallel about shoulder-width and press your palms beside your umbilicus. Extend the arms forward and lift them over the top of head. Straighten legs slowly at the same time. When hands reach the top, palms face forward. Look ahead. After a while, lean forward with legs extended. Draw the hands down along the Bladder Meridian. Lean the upper body forward when palms move downward along the back of legs to heels. Then move to the instep and pause for a moment. Do a massage from the lateral side of feet to medial side. Stretched the upper body and hands move upward along the inner thighs and reach beside the umbilicus. Repeat the process for 4-8 times. When you finish the last routine, slowly shift the weight downward. Knees are bent slightly. Arms rest beside the hip with palms facing downward and fingertips pointing forward. Look ahead.

1.7 Thrusting the Fists and Making the Eyes Glare to Enhance Strength

Squat down in a horse-riding stance. Hands are held in fist and positioned at the waist. Punch out slowly with left arm. Change palms and swivel arms. Stare at the distance with your left fist and pull your right fist back at the same time. Then draw the fist back to the waist. Relax your eyes and look ahead. Do the same routine to the right and repeat the whole process for 4-8 times. Finally, shift the weight rightward. Move the left leg back to stand with feet together. Unclench the fists and place hands naturally alongside the body. Look ahead.

1.8 Raising and Lowering the Heels to Cure Diseases

Stand naturally with feet together. Drop hands down naturally beside your body and look ahead. Raise up heels with straight back. Draw navel to spine and lift butt. Hold the posture for a few seconds before returning to the starting position. Repeat the bounce for 4-8 times, Inhale while lifting on both heels and exhale while returning. Relax the whole body. Finally, relax your whole body and breathe naturally. Sink *qi* down to *Dantian* and rest for a while.

2 Practice Tips

2.1 Combination of Relaxation, Coordination, Accuracy and Flexibility

Relaxation means having both mind and body relaxed in practice. Coordination indicates that the body, breath and mind should work coordinately. Accuracy mainly refers to proper posture and practice method. Flexibility signifies that adjustment should be made in movements range, posture height, used strength, exercises times, mentality and breathing according to one's own situation.

2.2　Combination of Training and Cultivation, and Step-by-step Practice

Training refers to a process where physical exercise, breathing adjustment and psychological adjustment are coordinated.

Cultivation is to reach a state where the body can rest queitly by relaxation and the mind in the natural condition through the above exercises.

The practicer should lay a solid foundation at the beginning of practice. Gradually correct postures are made. Actions are stretched with full spirit and energy, and become automatic.

第五章

中医养生与食疗
(Regimen and Dietary Therapy in Traditional Chinese Medicine)

中医养生是中医学的重要组成部分,是经过漫长实践与总结形成的以中医基础理论为指导、具备自身学术特点的养生观。养生是一种综合采用多方法、多途径、多措施,以自我保健为主要方式维持健康的行为,其中中医食疗是在中医理论的指导下利用食物的不同特性来改善人体功能的方法,兼具药食同源和五行养生的中医药特色优势。在健康中国背景下,中医养生与食疗的理念得到了社会的广泛认可和接受,且随着国家政策持续发力,推广中医养生与食疗对于传承中医文化,实现健康中国战略目标具有不可替代的作用。

Health Preservation is on important part of TCM. Its concept is guided by the basic theories of traditional Chinese medicine and has its own academic characteristics after a long period of practice and summary. Health preservation is a behavior that comprehensively adopts multiple methods, pathways, and measures, with self-care as the main way to maintain health. Traditional Chinese medicine diet therapy, guided by traditional Chinese medicine theory, utilizes the different characteristics of food to improve human body functions, and combines the unique advantages of the homology of medicine and food, the five-elements of nourishing health as well. Under the background of "Healthy China", the concept of the concept of health preservation and dietary therapy in traditional Chinese medicine has been widely recognized and accepted by society. With issuing the continuous national policies, the promotion of health preservation and dietary therapy in traditional Chinese medicine plays an irreplaceable role in inheriting traditional Chinese medicine culture and achieving the strategic goals of "Healthy China". This chapter will delve into the concepts, food characteristics, and dietary therapy methods of health preservation in traditional Chinese medicine, in order to fully develop its unique advantages health preservation and dietary therapy in traditional Chinese medicine. The traditional Chinese medicine culture represented is actively exporting in an international friendly environment, and becoming another powerful endorsement of China's image.

第一节　中医养生观念
（Concept of Regimen of Traditional Chinese Medicine）

中医养生观念源远流长，植根于中国古代哲学和中医基础理论。中医养生观念主要包括生命观、寿夭观、健康观、预防观、和谐观和权衡观。

一、生命观（View on Life）

（一）生命的物质观

生命是由物质化生，精、气、神是构成生命本质的要素。精是生命的物质基础，气是生命活动的动力，神是生命活动的主宰。三者协调统一，维持正常的生命状态。

1. 生命最基本的物质——精　精是构成人生命最基本的物质基础，是人生长发育及各种功能活动的物质基础。《素问·金匮真言论》云："精者，身之本也。"人的生命既来源于父母的先天之精，又受后天之精的濡养。而先天之精来源于父母，是生命形成的原始物质。《灵枢·决气》曰："两神相搏，合而成形，常先身生，是谓精。"万物化生皆从精始，男女之精相合构成了人之身形。先天之精在化生人体的过程中，一部分转化为脏腑之精，一部分封藏于肾。后天之精由水谷精微、外界吸入的清气以及各脏腑组织代谢化生的精微物质所组成，是维持生命的基础物质，是人出生后逐渐形成的。其中，水谷精微是后天之精的主要来源，而脾胃功能的强弱影响着后天之精的化生。先天之精与后天之精相互依存，共同为人体脏腑组织正常运行提供物质基础。

2. 生命的动力——气　气是指人体内活力很强、运行不息而无形可见的精微物质，是构成人体和维持人体生命活动的最基本物质。气是人体生命活动的动力。《难经·八难》曰："气者，人之根本也。"人的生命由天地间阴阳之气变化产生。气具有不断运动的特性，是人体生命活力的体现，具有推动、温煦、防御、固摄、气化、营养的作用。同时，气也表示脏腑组织的功能活动。人体一身之气分布于不同的部位，具有不同的生理作用，据此命名为不同的气。如一身之气分布于人体五脏，则称为五脏之气；气分布于六腑，则称为六腑之气；气分布于经络，则称为经络之气等。

3. 生命活动的主宰——神　神是对人体生命活动外在表现的高度概括，是生命活动的主宰。《素问·移精变气论》云："得神者昌，失神者亡。"通过神的盛衰，可以判定人体的健康状况与疾病的轻重及预后。生命活动正常，神表现旺盛，称为有神；生命活动异常，神表现为不足，称为少神；生命活动衰微，神出现衰败，称为失神，表示病情严重，预后不良。因此，神健则形体充，疾病不侵；神不足则气弱，易于致病。摄神，调神为养生的第一要义。神主宰人的精神意识、思想活动，神包括魂、魄、意、志、思、虑等。神调则七情平和,魂魄内守,机体内部脏腑功能协调,气血畅达,营卫通利。

精、气、神是组成生命的基本要素,是密不可分的统一整体,精充、气足、神旺是生命充满活力的根本保证。精为气的物质基础,气为精的生命力表现,在精与气的相互转化中显现出人体的各种生理活动,故将两者合称为精气,精与气是神的物质基础。精、气、神三者在生理上相互联系,病理上相互影响,它们相互协调,共同维持正常的人体生命活动。

（二）生命的运动变化观

万物具有永恒运动的特性。升、降、出、入是气的基本运动形式,同时也是脏腑、经络及组织器官运动的基本过程。气的升降出入运动,推动和激发着人体的各项生理活动,气的升降出入协调平衡,人体则可保持正常的生理活动;若气的升降出入平衡失常,人体便会出现各种病理状态;气的升降出入一旦停止,意味着生命活动的终止。

二、寿夭观（View on Lifetime）

寿夭是指人体生长发育衰老的状况。寿,是指能尽终其天年、自然衰老而逝者;夭,是指不及天年、早衰而亡者。寿者身心健康,年益寿延;夭者形神不保,病多寿折。天年是指天赋的年寿,即自外寿命。人的生命是有一定期限的,古代医家、养生家认为人的寿命在百岁到一百二十岁之间。先天禀赋和后天因素决定了人寿命的长短和衰老的进程。

（一）先天禀赋

先天禀赋的强弱对人寿命的长短和衰老的进程有着重要的影响。先天禀赋指子代出生以前在母体内所禀受的一切,包括父母精血之强弱、父母血缘的遗传性、在胎育过程中是否有疾病或药物损伤等。先天禀赋强,则身体强壮,精力充沛,不易衰老;先天禀赋弱,则身体虚弱,精神萎靡,病多夭。

父母体质是先天禀赋的决定因素。《幼科发挥》曰:"夫男女之生,受气于父,成形于母。故父母强者,生子亦强,父母弱者,生子亦弱,所以肥瘦、长短、大小、妍媸,皆肖父母也。"父母双方应该尽量在健康的状态下生儿育女。母亲胎育的过程也会影响胎儿的禀赋,胎孕期间应注重保养。此外,先天禀赋不足、先天禀赋不纯、先天禀赋残缺都会对机体带来很大影响,导致后天气血失调,明阳失和而化生疑难之症。

（二）后天因素

后天因素对人寿命的长短以及衰老的进程也有着重要的影响。后天因素主要包括行为方式、疾病损伤、自然环境及社会环境。

1.行为方式　行为方式包括饮食、起居、劳逸、嗜好等。良好适度的行为方式有利于健康,不良的行为方式会导致疾病的发生。顺应天地阴阳的变化,饮食有节制,起居有规律,不过分劳作,则可尽享天年,反之则损害健康。现代研究报告也指出,吸烟、过量饮酒、身体活动不足和不健康饮食是慢性疾病发生及发展的主要危险因素。

2.疾病损伤　疾病与健康共同存在于生命过程中。疾病损害健康,促进衰老。不同时代引起人口死亡的主要原因不尽相同。目前我国居民的生活方式、饮食结构、环境状况等发生了实质性的变化,尤其是人口城市化、老龄化、环境污染和生活方式的变化使我国人口的疾病模式也发生了变化,慢性疾病已成为导致我国人口死亡的主要原因。据《中国居民营养与慢性疾病状况报告(2020年)》指出:"2019年我国因慢性疾病导致的死亡占总死亡88.5%。其中心脑血管病、癌症、慢性呼吸系统疾病死亡比例为80.7%。"因此,应预防疾病发生,遏制疾病加重。

3.自然环境　自然环境与人寿命长短和衰老进程有着密切的联系。自然环境是指影响人类的各种自然因素的总和,包括地形地貌、大气、水、土壤、岩石矿物、太阳辐射等。地域差异的大小和人的寿夭有着密切的关系,地域差异小,寿夭的差别小;地域差异大,寿夭的差别就大。现代由于工业的发展及人类对自然的过度索取,导致地球生态破坏、资源短缺、环境污染,人类的健康遭受了极大的威胁。如严重空气污染造成的雾霾天气会损伤呼吸系统,易诱发心血管疾病的急性发作,还会影响儿童的生长发育。人类应保护环境,采取积极措施应对环境污染带来的危害。

4.社会环境　社会环境对人的寿夭有着重要的影响。构成社会环境的相关因素包括政治因素、经济因素、文化因素等。社会环境安定,人们才得以安居乐业,颐养天年;反之,社会环境动荡、战火纷飞,人们的生命安全得不到保障,生活的基本物质需求得不到满足,长期处于恐慌、焦虑的情绪中,健康必然会受到严重的影响。目前中国大规模的城市化、持续的工业化、快速的经济发展带来了激烈的社会竞争,高强度的工作、生活压力对人们的健康造成了极大的影响。

三、健康观（View on Health）

健康观指人们对健康的认识,医学最终的目的和意义是维护人类的健康,正确的健康观是人们进行养生保健活动的基础。由于中西医学体系的不同,对于健康的认识和理解有所差异,现将中医健康观和以西方医学为基础的现代健康观阐述如下。

（一）中医健康观

中医健康观一直以来内容较为丰富,体现了中医对健康深刻的认识和理解。中医健康观包括"天人合一"的健康观、"形神合一"的健康观、"阴平阳秘"的健康观、"正气为本"的健康观等。藏象、经络、病因、病机等中医学理论的主要内容都是围绕着中医健康观而展开。医学将健康的人称为"平人",《素问·调经论》曰:"阴阳匀平,以充其形,九候若一,命曰平人。"健康的人应包括身体健康、心理健康,同时还与自然、社会的变化协调平衡。此外,道德健康也是健康的重要内容,在社会交往中不慕高贵,不鄙卑微,真诚质朴,才能脏腑气血调和,达到身体的健康。

(二)现代健康观

现代医学根植于西方医学。早在古希腊时期,西方医学之父希波克拉底认为通过保持土、火、风、水四元素的平衡即可保持健康,并认为机体应与外界环境相协调。随着细胞的发现、解剖学的兴起,西方医学走上了一条不断探索人体各部分的形态和结构的道路,开始重视躯体结构、生理功能的健康。随着社会的发展,现代的医学模式已经由单纯的"生物医学"转变为"生物-心理-社会医学"。1989 年世界卫生组织提出了 21 世纪健康新概念:"健康,不仅是没有疾病,而且包括躯体健康、社会适应良好和道德健康。"人类对健康的认识又深入了一步,健康的概念由生物健康的领域扩充到了社会健康的领域。

综上所述,中医健康观与现代健康观具有一致性,体现了中医健康理念的前瞻性与科学性。在治疗疾病的过程中,现代医学逐渐重视对患者思维意识活动、生存质量的疗效评价,更加注意患者的三观感受,提高患者舒适度,改善患者的心情及痛苦程度。较之于现代医学,中医在诊治患者时更加重视患者的就医愿望。一些患者在就诊时存在躯体的不适或痛苦,经现代医学检查并未见明显异常,但通过中医四诊合参、辨证论治,可解除患者的不适,实现患者的就医愿望。

四、预防观(View on Prevention)

中医预防观的核心观点为"治未病",最早见于《黄帝内经》。中医所指"未病",有两层含义:第一层含义为"尚无病"时的未病,主要针对健康人群和亚健康人群;第二层含义为"已病"状态下的未病,主要针对已患有疾病的人。中医"治未病"主要从以下 4 个方面进行阐述。

(一)未病先防,养生保全

未病先防是指人体在没有发生疾病的健康或亚健康状态下,预先采取养生保健措施,目的在于固护正气,提高身体素质,祛病延年,健康益寿。古代医家提出了一些未病先防的方法。中医养生学通过清心养性、节欲保精、顺应四时、因地制宜、饮食调养、导引吐纳等方法,均可达到未病先防、养生保全的目的。

(二)欲病早治,防微杜渐

《素问·刺热》云:"肝热病者左颊先赤,心热病者颜先赤,脾热病者鼻先赤,肺热病者右颊先赤,肾热病者颐先赤。病虽未发,见赤色者刺之,名曰治未病。"此为"治未病"的第二层含义,是指中医对功能调整的优势,采取多种手段和方法促使"欲病"向健康转化。有效预防的关键在于懂得谨小慎微、仔细观察,在疾病典型症状出现之前就能观察到发病的先兆,先给予适当的治疗,使之不发病,避免疾病的困扰,如强忍不治,认为可自愈,过些时日则可发为顽固之疾。

（三）审因察势，已病防变

分析疾病发生发展的趋势，通过辨证求因，进行有针对性的预防，此为"治未病"的第三层含义。《金匮要略·脏腑经络先后病脉证》谓："问曰，上工治未病，何也？师曰，夫治未病者，见肝之病，知肝传脾，当先实脾。四季脾土不受邪，即勿补之。中工不晓相传，见肝之病，不解实脾，治肝也。"人体的表里内外、五脏六腑、经络气血是相互联系的，病变可遵循规律进行防治。

（四）祛邪务尽，病后防复

疾病经治疗后，病邪已基本消除，正气尚未恢复，此时应谨防疾病复发。可采取以下措施防止疾病的复发：疾病初愈、余邪未清时，应积极扶助正气，继续清除余邪；不应过于劳累，以防劳复；由于脾胃运化能力尚弱，应当节制饮食，不宜进食辛辣生冷及不易消化的食物，以防食复；人体元气未复，应当节房事，养肾精，以防房复；情志过激会伤及脏腑，应当调和情志，调养心神，以防因情复病。

五、和谐观（View on Harmony）

和谐观是中国传统文化的核心理念。宇宙万物是阴阳二气相合的统一体。《广韵》载："和，顺也；谐也，不坚不柔也。"和谐，可解释为调和、和解、生化、促进，以及使之平和、使之平衡、使之协调、使之有序、使之顺畅、使之适度、使之舒展、使之条达等。

中医学的理论和实践处处渗透着和谐的观点，包括对人体生理功能的认识和理解，对疾病治疗的方法与手段，都以协调和平衡为核心。健康状态是一种人体各脏腑组织之间、人体与外部环境之间相和谐的状态。人体"和"的状态即为健康的状态，包括"血和""卫气和""志意和""寒温和"。中医的整体观念是中医和谐观的高度概括，强调人与自然、人与社会、人体本身内部脏器之间的和谐。阴阳五行学说强调人体内部各脏腑组织之间相互依存、相互制约、处于一种协调和谐的状态，和谐一旦被打破则产生疾病。平衡阴阳、协调脏腑、调和气血等中医治法都是以恢复人体的和谐为目的，所以和谐观也是中医学的核心理念。

六、权衡观（View on *Quanheng*）

权衡原义为称量物体轻重的器具。权，秤砣；衡，秤杆。司马迁《史记》载："平权衡，正度量，调轻重。"权衡更深层的意义是指事物在动态中维持平衡的状态。中医的权衡观把人体脏腑组织之间动态平衡的调节过程以及人体与外界环境之间动态平衡的调节过程比作"权"与"衡"的关系。为维持动态平衡的状态，人体脏腑组织之间、人体与外环境之间不断增减移动，进行调节。中医养生学的权衡观是指通过权衡以养护生命，维持人体生命常态，从而达到健康长寿的目的。当人体出现阴阳失衡，气血不畅时，应因势利导,补正纠偏,使人体达到阴平阳秘、气血和畅、精神内的状态。中医养生学的权衡观主要体现在以下几方面。

（一）权衡情志

中医学认为人是"形与神俱"的生命统一体,神者,生之本也,神不调则脏腑不和。狭义的"神"即指人的情志活动。适度而有节制的情志活动对机体的生理功能起着协调的作用;反之,持久强烈的情志变化超过了人体的生理和心理适应能力,会导致气机失调、阴阳失衡、脏腑功能紊乱。因此,应通过权衡情志来养神,可采用修身养性、疏泄情绪、移情易性、以情胜情、四时调神等方法,使情志无太过和不及,使人体达到平衡协调、阴平阳秘的状态。

（二）权衡饮食

饮食是人体赖以生存和维持健康的物质基础,不合理的饮食习惯、饮食方式是引起疾病的重要原因。在日常生活中应做到饮食有节,五味调和,注意饮食宜忌,使体内营养均衡、脏腑功能稳定。应避免饥饱失常、饮食偏嗜、饮食不洁等情况的发生。过饥则气血生化无源,无以濡养人体脏腑组织;过饱则影响脾胃运化水谷的功能,日久则助湿、化热、生痰而产生疾病。权衡饮食的关键在于食物的搭配、食味的调和。食物搭配是指日常的食物要有多样性,应全面摄取人体所需的各种营养成分,应注意各类食物所占的比例,荤素的搭配、粗粮和细粮的搭配要合理。食味的调和是指食物具有酸、苦、甘、辛、咸 5 种不同的性味,当食物组合在一起时性味要相协调。

（三）权衡劳逸

《管子·形势》曰:"起居时,饮食节,寒暑适,则身利而寿命益。起居不时,饮食不节,寒暑不适,则形体累而寿命损。"中医养生理论认为,饮食起居有规律,劳逸结合,顺应昼夜阴阳消长的变化,顺应四时生、长、化、收、藏的规律,就能保养神气,避免疾病的发生,达到健康长寿的目的。在日常生活中应权衡劳逸进行养生,每天都需要适度的活动,才可以振奋阳气、通畅气血,脏腑组织才能正常运行。劳逸失常会引发疾病,如果过度劳累,则消耗精气,损伤气血;如果过度安逸,则气血郁滞,脏腑功能减退。

The time-honored concept of health cultivation of TCM is rooted in ancient Chinese philosophy and basic theory of TCM. It includes views on life, on lifetime, on fitness, on the prevention of diseases, on harmony and on *quanheng* (weighing).

1 View on Life

1.1 Life Is Essentially Material

Life comes from substance, with essence, *qi*, spirit being its basic ingredients. The material basis of life is the essence. And life activities are promoted by *qi* and governed by spirit. The three coordinately maintain a normal life state.

1.1.1　The Most Fundamental Substance of Life—Essence

The essence is the most basic substance to constitute the human body, which serves as the material basis of human growth, development, and various functional activities. As is described in the *Jinkui Zhenyan Lun* of *Su Wen* (*Discussion on Important Ideas in the Golden Chamber*, the chapter of *Plain Conversation*), "essence is the foundation of the body". Human life is derived from congenital essence and nourished by acquired essence. Inherited from parents, the congenital essence is primitive substance that forms the life. In the *Jueqi* of *Ling Shu* (*Differentiation of Qi*, the chapter of *Spiritual Pivot*), it is described that "when two spirits are interacting on each other, the reproductive essence of a male and female combines to conceive a fetus. The reproductive substance that exists before the conception of the fetus is called *jing* (essence)." All the beings start from essence. It is the combination of male's and female's essence that forms human body. When transforming the body, a part of congenital essence is changed into the essence of *zang-fu* organs, and others is stored in kidney. The acquired essence consists of nutrients absorbed from food and water, clear *qi* inhaled from external environment and substance transformed via *zang-fu* organs metabolism, which gradually forms after one's birth and sustains one's life. Among them, the nutrients of food and water is the major source. And whether the spleen and stomach can function well makes a difference to the transformation of the acquired essence. The two interdependent kinds of essence play a vital role in helping *zang-fu* organs function normally.

1.1.2　The Engine of Life—*Qi*

Qi refers to the energetic, intangible and subtle substances that move constantly through the human body, which plays a crucial part in constituting human body and maintaining its life activity. It serves as an engine of human life activities. This is why *Nan Jing* (*Classic of Difficulties*) states that "vital energy is the root of human being". Life generates from *yin qi* and *yang qi* in the universe. Characterized by constant motion, *qi* manifests vitality, which has the function of propelling, warming, defending, consolidating, transforming and nourishing. Also, *qi* refers to functional activities of viscera. The *qi* in different parts of human body has different psychological function and is named accordingly. For example, the *qi* distributed in five *zang-*organs is called the *qi* of *zang-*organs. The *qi* in six *fu-*organs is called the *qi* of *fu-*organs, and the *qi* in meridians is called the *qi* of meridians.

1.1.3　The Dominator of Life Activities—Spirit

Spirit highly generalizes the external manifestation of life activity, and governs it. In the *Yijing Bianqi Lun* of *Su Wen* (*Discussion on Shifting the Essence and Changing the Qi*, the chapter of *Plain Conversation*), it is described that "loss of spirit causes death while maintenance of spirit ensures life". It means that the observation of one's spirit can help assess health condition, the severity of disease and prognosis. *Youshen* refers to normal life activity and sufficient spirit. *Shaoshen* indicates insufficiency of spirit. *Shishen* refers to weak life activities and exhaustion of spirit, a sign indicating the worsen disease and poor prognosis. Therefore, adequate spirit brings on a powerful physique without invasion of diseases while inadequate spirit results in deficiency of *qi* and predisposition to disease, so it should be taken as priority to cultivate and regulate spirit in health preservation. Spirit governs spiritual awareness and mental activity of human being, including soul, corporeal soul, consciousness, will, contemplation, consideration and so on. A harmonized spirit can keep seven emotions normal and soul intact, and ensures normal function of viscera, free flow of *qi* and blood as well as smoothness of *Ying*-nutrients and *Wei*-defensive.

Essence, *qi* and spirit are basic elements that constitute life, which are inseparable and should be seen as a unity. It is the sufficiency of these substances that ensures a vibrant life. Essence is the material basis of *qi*, and in turn, is manifested by it. Since they transform into each other in various physiological activities of human body, they are often put together and called *jingqi*. Besides, essence and *qi* are material basis of spirit. Physiologically and pathologically interrelated, the three coordinate with each other to maintain normal life activities.

1.2　Life Is in Constant Motion

Everything is in eternal motion. *Qi* movement is manifested in such basic forms as ascending, descending, exiting and entering, which is also the basic process of the movement of viscera, meridians and organs. It motivates and propels the various physiological activities of human body. That means if *qi* moves in balance, physiological activities will run their course. However, unbalanced movement of *qi* will result in all kinds of pathological conditions. Once it stops, life will come to an end.

2　View on Lifetime

Shouyao refers to the growth, development and aging of human body. *Shou* refers to those who live a long and healthy life, while *yao* refers to those who cannot live as long as their life span expects. *Tiannian* means lifespan. Human life is limited and one is expected to live for 100-120 years according to ancient physicians and health practitioners. Life expectancy and aging are determined by congenital endowment and acquired factors.

2.1　Congenital Endowment

Congenital endowment has an important impact on life expectancy and aging. It refers to what babies received before birth, including essence, heredity, or drug damage during pregnancy, etc. It can be said that the baby with strong endowment is robust and energetic, and ages slowly; the one with weak endowment is feeble and listless.

Whether the baby can have strong endowment depends on parents' constitution. As is described in *Youke Fahui* (*Elaborations on Pediatric Treatments*), "the new life inherits *qi* from father and comes into being in the uterus of mother. Therefore, healthy parents will give birth to healthy children and vice versa. Children, fat or thin, tall or short, beautiful or ugly, look like their parents". It means that parents should be both in good health if they want to have children. Also, what mothers do during pregnancy will have an effect on fetus' endowment, thus pregnant mothers should pay attention to take good care of health. Additionally, insufficiency or impurity of congenital endowment will give rise to diseases due to disharmony between *qi* and blood, *yin* and *yang* in human body.

2.2 Acquired Factors

Acquired factors also exert an important effect on life expectancy and aging, mainly including behavior, impair, disease as well as natural and social environment.

2.2.1 Behavior

It refers to eating and living, work and rest, hobbies, etc. Good behavior is conducive to health while bad behavior can lead to diseases. Adapting to the changing *yin* and *yang* in the universe, those who have a balanced diet and regular living habits without overwork will live a long life, otherwise it will damage health. Furthermore, modern research shows that the main factors accounting for the occurrence and development of chronic diseases include smoking, excessive drinking, lack of exercise and unhealthy diet.

2.2.2 Impair and Disease

Disease and health coexist in the course of life. Disease damages health and accelerates aging. People in different eras die from different causes. Currently, there emerges substantial changes in Chinese residents' lifestyle, diet and environmental conditions. In particular, the disease pattern changes because of population urbanization, aging, environmental pollution and new lifestyle, thus making chronic disease become the main cause of death in China. According to the *Report on Chinese Nutrition and Chronic Diseases* (*2020*), "deaths caused by chronic diseases accounted for 88.5% of total deaths in China in 2019. Cardiovascular and cerebrovascular diseases, cancer and chronic respiratory diseases accounted for 80.7% of the deaths". Therefore, it is necessary to prevent the occurrence and aggravation of the disease.

2.2.3 Natural Environment

Natural environment is closely related to life span and aging process. Natural environment refers to various natural factors influencing human beings, including topography, atmosphere, water, soil, rocks, minerals, solar radiation. There is a close relationship between regions and longevity. Great regional differences lead to huge differences in longevity. Nowadays, human beings are facing health challenges caused by the ecosystem destruction, resource shortage and environmental pollution due to industrial development and the unrestrained exploitation of natural resources. For example, being exposed to the fog and thick haze that are caused by serious air pollution will damage the respiratory system, induce acute cardiovascular diseases and affect children's growth. As a result, it is necessary that humans take an active part in environmental conservation.

2.2.4 Social Environment

Social environment has an important influence on longevity. It includes political, economic, cultural factors. A stable society enables people to live and work in peace and contentment and to enjoy natural lifespan. Contrarily, a society in turbulence and wars neither meet people's basic need, nor guarantee their safety, where people absolutely suffer from health problems for living in a long-term panic and anxiety. Additionally, people's health is also affected by fierce social competition and high intensity work and life pressure brought by the current large-scale urbanization, ongoing industrialization and rapid economic development in China.

3　View on Health

The view on health refers to people's understanding of health. The ultimate goal of medicine is to maintain health and that's why it exists. A positive view on health is important for people to keep healthy, but views on it vary because of the differences between Chinese and western medical system. The health view of TCM and the modern health view based on western medicine are elaborated as follows.

3.1　The TCM View on Health

The concept of health in TCM, always rich in contents, embodies the profound knowledge and understanding of health. It includes views of harmony between man and nature, unity of body and spirit, balance between *yin* and *yang* as well as harmony. Theories of viscera manifestation, meridians, etiology and pathogenesis are all based on the health concept of TCM. A healthy person is called *pingren*, as it is stated in *Tiaojing Lun* of *Su Wen* (*Discussion on the Regualtion of Channels*, the chapter of *Plain Conversation*) that " *yin* and *yang* are balanced, the body is sufficiently nourished and the pulse states in the nine divisions are the same. This is *pingren* (the normal condition of a man)". A fit person should be in good health both physically and mentally and meanwhile strike a balance between nature, society and himself. In addition, moral health is also an important part of health. Not being snobbish and being sincere and simple are what we should do in social interaction. Only by this can we harmonize the qi and blood of viscera, thus maintaining a good health.

3.2 The Modern View on Health

Modern medicine is rooted in western medicine. It was early in the ancient Greece that Hippocrates, the father of western medicine, believed that striking the balance of earth, fire, wind and water was necessary to maintain health and that the body should be in harmony with the external environment. With the discovery of cells and the rise of anatomy, western medicine embarked on a path toward the constant exploration of the form and structure of each part of the human body, and began to pay attention to body structure and physiological function. With the development of society, the modern medical model has changed from simple "biomedical" to "bio-psycho-social medicine". In 1989, the World Health Organization put forward a new concept of health in the 21st century: "Health is a complete state of physical, mental and social well-being, and not merely the absence of disease or infirmity. " That means a further understanding of health as humans explore it from a biological aspect to a social perspective.

To conclude, the concept of health in TCM is consistent with the modern view of health, which reflects the forward-looking and scientific nature of the health notion of TCM. In the process of treating diseases, modern medicine gradually attaches importance to the curative effect evaluation of patients' mental activity and life quality, and pays more attention to patients' three-way feelings, improves patients' comfortability and mood as well as alleviates the pain. Compared with it, TCM focuses more on patients' desire for medical treatment. Some patients feel uncomfortable or painful, but no obvious abnormality can be found through modern medical examination. However, the symptoms can be relieved by the combination of four diagnostic methods and the treatment based on syndrome differentiation, thus realizing the patients' desire.

4 View on Prevention

Zhi Weibing (prevention treatment) is at the core of prevention view of TCM, which was first seen in *Huangdi Neijing*. There are two meanings of *Weibing* in TCM. One is *Weibing* before a disease arises, mainly for healthy and sub-healthy people; the other is that after the onset of the disease, mainly for people suffering from illnesses. It will be elaborated from the following four aspects.

4.1 Preventing Before a Disease Arises and Preserving Health

Prevention before a disease arises means that the humans take proactive measures to maintain health when they are in a healthy or sub-healthy state, aiming at consolidating the healthy *qi*, improving physical fitness, curing diseases and prolonging life. Ancient physicians put forward some methods of preventing diseases before they occur. Health cultivation in TCM holds that prevention before a disease arises and health preservation can be achieved by maintaining a tranquil mind, storing essence by abstinence, adapting to seasonal changes and local conditions, keeping a balanced diet and taking breathing exercises.

4.2　Treating the Disease as Early as Possible Against Its Development

As is stated in *Cire* of *Su Wen* (*Discussion on Acupuncture Treatment* of *Febrile Diseases*, the chapter of *Plain Conversation*) , "In the febrile disease of the liver, the left cheek turns red first; in the febrile disease of the heart, the forehead turns red first; in the febrile disease of the spleen, the nose turns red first; in the febrile disease of the lung, the right cheek turns red first; in the febrile disease of the kidney, the *yi* (the lateral part inferior to the mouth corner) turns red first. Acupuncture can be used when certain part of the face turns red, though the disease has not occurred yet. Such a way of treatment is known as to treat diseases in advance. This is the second meaning of *Zhi Weibing*" , which refers to the advantages of traditional Chinese medicine in adjusting functions. It adopts various means and methods to help people prevent diseases and become healthy. The key to effective prevention lies in careful observation. Before the typical symptoms of the disease appear, appropriate treatment is necessary after the precursor is observed, by which the disease can be avoided so people will not suffer from it. If we ignore it, thinking that we can heal ourselves, the disease will become difficult to treat in a few days.

4.3　Preventing Transmission of a Disease After its Onset by Examining Its Cause and Tendency

It is the third meaning of "*Zhi Weibing*" to analyze the disease tendency and to carry out targeted prevention based on syndrome differentiation. It is described in *Jinkui Yaolue* (*Synopsis of Golden Chamber*) that "Question: Would you kindly explain the meaning of ' A superior doctor will cure a disease before its onset? ' Master: ' To cure a disease before its onset' means that when the Liver is affected, a prescription is chosen to replenish the Spleen, as the doctor knows the Liver disease will be transmitted into the Spleen. During the last periods of each season, the Spleen Vital Energy is strong enough to resist transmission of the pathogenic factors, so the Spleen does not need to be replenished. A mediocre doctor would not know about the transmission. So he would not replenish the Spleen when the Liver is affected. " There is an interrelation between the exterior and interior, external and internal, five *zang* – organs and six *fu* –

organs, meridians and *qi* and blood, so pathological changes can be prevented and treated based on that.

4. 4 Eliminating Evil Factors Thoroughly to Prevent the Relapse

The pathogenic factors have been almost eliminated after treatment, but the healthy *qi* has not been restored. Hence, we should prevent the recurrence of the disease at this point. The following measures can be taken to prevent the relapse: when the recovery is at an initial stage and there are still pathogens in the body, we should actively cultivate the healthy *qi* and continue to eliminate the left pathogens. Do not overwork. Have a balanced diet and avoid eating food that is spicy, raw, cold and indigestible due to the weakness of transportation and transformation of the spleen and stomach. Reduce sexual intercourse to nourish kidney essence as the primordial *qi* is not restored. Maintain emotional stability and nourish the mind as being overly emotional will do harm to the viscera. All of these is to prevent relapse.

5 View on Harmony

The view on harmony is the key concept of Chinese traditional culture. Everything in the universe can be seen as a unity of *yin* and *yang*. According to the rhyme dictionary *Guangyun* (*Extened Ryhmes*), "*He* can be interpreted as smoothness and harmony, not being overly firm or soft". He Xie(Harmony) also has the same meaning of regulation, reconciliation, transformation and promotion as well as gentleness, balance, coordination, order, smoothness, moderation, stretch and free development.

The view on harmony exerts a great influence on the theory and practice of TCM, including the understanding of human physiological functions and treatment method of disease, all of which take coordination and balance as the core. Being healthy refers to a state with harmony between viscera and tissues, human body and external environment. The state of "harmony" in human body indicates one is healthy, including harmony in blood, *Wei*-defence and *qi*, emotion and mind as well as well-adaption to coldness and warmness. The holistic concept of TCM highly generalizes the view on harmony, which emphasizes the harmony between man and nature, man and society, and internal organs within human body. The theory of *yin* and *yang* and Five-Elements lay stress on a harmonious state between the *zang-fu* organs and tissues of the human body that are interdependent and mutually restricted. Diseases will occur once the harmony is broken. TCM treating methods such as balancing yin and yang, coordinating viscera and harmonizing *qi* and blood are all aimed at restoring the harmony in human body, so it can be said that the view on harmony is also the key concept of traditional Chinese medicine.

6 View on *Quanheng*

Quanheng originally refers to weighing apparatus, with *quan* being the weight and *heng* being the steelyard. It is stated in *Shiji* (*Records of the Grand Historian*) written by *Sima Qian* that "unified measures for length, capacity and weight". Also, it is, in a further sense, a state in which things are kept in a dynamic balance. In the view on *quanheng* of TCM, there is dynamic balance between viscera, between human body and external environment. So there will be increment and subtraction as well as movement between the viscera and tissues, and between human body and the external environment in adjustment to maintain the dynamic balance. The view on *quanheng* in health preservation in TCM holds that people should maintain their life by *quanheng* to keep the normal state of life, so that they can live a healthy and long life. When *yin* and *yang* are out of balance, and *qi* and blood cannot flow smoothly, we should make timely corrections according to circumstances, in an effort to return the balance between *yin* and *yang*, and harmony in *qi* and blood as well as maintain the spirit. The view is mainly reflected in the following aspects.

6.1 Emotions

TCM holds that human life is the unity of body and spirit. As spirit is the foundation of life, it will incur the dysfunction of viscera if the spirit is improperly regulated. In a narrow sense, spirit refers to mental activities. Moderate mental activities play an integral role in coordinating physiological functions of the body. On the contrary, persistent and strong emotional changes, which go beyond the physiological and psychological adaptability of human body, will lead to impediment of *qi* movement, imbalance of *yin* and *yang* and disorder of viscera. Therefore, the spirit should be nourished by *quanheng*, including self – cultivation, catharsis, removal of bad mood by suppressing it with another emotion, spirits regulation in light of seasonal changes, so that emotions are kept in moderate range, which helps to achieve the balance between *yin* and *yang*.

6.2 Diet

Diet provides the material basis for human body to survive and maintain health. Unreasonable eating habits and ways are main causes of diseases. In daily life, we should have a balanced diet in harmony of five flavors. The balanced nutrition helps viscera function in stability. We should avoid over-hunger, overeating, dietary bias and unclean diet. Being famished leads to the lack of resource of generating and transforming *qi* and blood, failing to nourish viscera and tissues, while overeating affects transformation of nutrients performed by spleen and stomach, which will cause diseases by producing dampness, heat and phlegm if left untreated. The most crucial part is the collocation of food and the harmony of tastes. The former refers to a diversified diet in daily life. It is important to intake all kinds of nutrients that human body needs. The proportion of various foods, and the collocation of meat and vegetables, coarse grains and fine grains should be reasonable. The latter means that the taste of sour, bitter, sweet, pungent and salty should be coordinated in food combination.

6.3 Work and Rest

According to *Xingshi* of *Guanzi* (*Conditions and Circumstances*, the chapter of *The Book of Master Guan*), "it is conducive to health and prolong life to have regular work and rest, balanced diet and well-adaptation to seasonal changes. Otherwise, it will damage health. " TCM holds that regular eating and living, alternate work with rest, conform to the changes of *yin* and *yang* in day and night, as well as the laws of birth, growth, transformation, harvest and storage in four seasons. The spirit can be nourished and diseases avoided so that people can live a healthy and long life. In daily life, we should preserve health by striking a balance between work and rest. Take exercises every day to invigorate *yang qi*, and smooth *qi* and blood, so that viscera and tissues can work as normal. Unbalance between work and rest will cause diseases. Overwork will consume essence and damage *qi* and blood, while idleness brings about stagnated *qi* and blood as well as viscera hypofunction.

第二节　四季养生
(Regimen in Four Seasons)

人们生活在天地之间,天人相应,应当遵循自然界气候变化的规律,才能有助于维护机体健康。若自然界的气候变化违背常规,出现异常情况,在天人相应的影响下人也会受到一定程度的影响,甚至影响健康。《伤寒论》记载:"春气温和,夏气暑热,秋气清凉,冬气冰冽,此四时正气之序也。"这是自然界正常的气候变化规律。在正常气候变化规律下,人体如果发病,也会一定程度上体现正常气候变化的特点。如《素问·金匮真言论》载:"春善病鼽衄,仲夏善病胸胁,长夏善病洞泄寒中,秋善病风疟,冬善病痹厥。"《伤寒论》又载:"凡时行者,春时应暖而反大寒,夏时应热而反大凉,秋时应凉而反大热,冬时应寒而反大温,此非其时而有其气。是以一岁之中,长幼之病多相似者,此则时行之气也。"说明如果气候变化违背常规,出现"非其时而有其气"的情况,就会发生症状表现相似的病症,经常是由"非其时而有其气"导致。

一、春季养生(Regimen in Spring)

春季从立春之日起,到立夏之日止,包括立春、雨水、惊蛰、春分、清明、谷雨6个节气。春为四季之首,立春是一年中的第一个节气。《素问·四气调神大论》有:"春三月,此谓发陈。天地俱生,万物以荣。"描述了春回大地,阳气升发,自然界生机勃勃、欣欣向荣的景象。春应五脏之肝,属木,春季也是肝气条畅之际。从生理角度讲,春温春生,春季人体阳气升发于外,人们在起居调摄、精神、饮食、运动等方面都应该顺应春天阳气升发、万物始生的特点,保养"生发"之气。

春季养生中,要注意阳气的升发和肝气的调畅,在起居方面要入夜睡眠,天明起床免冠披发,松带宽衣,以舒展身体的气机和形体。衣着方面,即便天气转温,也不应快速减衣,特别是年老体弱者以及有基础疾病的人群,减脱冬装应谨慎,不可骤减,符合春捂秋冻;春季应注意精神情志疾病的复发,可以采用多种方式方法,促进心胸开阔,保持愉快的精神状态,如踏青、吟诵等都可陶冶情操,调畅机体有助于放松精神,保持情绪平稳乐观。春季宜食辛甘发散之品而不宜食酸收之味,如韭菜、大葱、洋葱、生姜等有助于养阳升阳;春季气候逐渐变暖,衣物也随温度的升高而逐渐减少,身体负担逐渐减轻。前往空气清新之处、登山、赏花都是春季运动养生不错的选择,但需注意不可运动过量,过犹不及致身体疲惫不堪。运动前要检查衣物是否合适,鞋子一定要有弹性,穿透气鞋袜。心脑血管疾病患者选择运动时要注意符合自身健康状况,不可争强好胜。

二、夏季养生(Regimen in Summer)

夏季从立夏之日起,至立秋之日止,包括立夏、小满、芒种、夏至、小暑、大暑6个节气,是一年之中阳气最旺盛的季节。《素问·四气调神大论》有:"夏三月,此谓蕃秀。天地气交,万物华实。"夏季万物繁茂秀美,阳气旺盛,是长养万物的季节,是阳极阴生、万物成熟的季节。夏应五脏之心,属火。夏热夏长,从生理角度讲,夏季机体阳气也旺于外,夏季养生要顺应夏季阳盛于外的特点,注意养护阳气,着眼于"养长",五脏重在养心。此外,长夏多湿多雨,天地之间湿热蒸腾,与五脏之脾相应,然而脾喜燥恶湿,因而此时最易伤脾,故长夏养生应重视健脾。

在酷暑季节,白天应减少剧烈活动,多去阴凉之处避暑,外出戴太阳帽、打遮阳伞、戴太阳镜等。盛夏季节出汗较多,应勤洗澡、勤换衣,保持皮肤和衣物洁净;夏季气候炎热,易心浮气躁,而保持平和的心态及愉悦心情有益于减轻燥热感,听舒缓音乐、喝绿茶、练习书法等对于保持心境有一定的帮助;在炎热夏季,易导致寒气入肺而伤肺,可适当食用辛味的食物如萝卜、葱白、姜蒜、韭苔等,但不可多吃。夏季腠理开泄,汗出较多,可酌情食用酸味食物,有助于收敛肌腠,同时可以生津止渴,例如酸梅汤;夏季运动时要注意避光避暑,避免在日照强烈温度最高的正午运动,防止中暑,最好在清晨或傍晚较凉爽时运动,运动场地可选择公园、庭院、水边等空气清新之处,夏天不宜做剧烈的运动,防止出现汗泄太过耗气伤津的情况,游泳、散步、慢跑、太极拳、广播操等运动量较为适宜。运动过程中注意补水,运动后不要立即用冷水冲头淋浴。

三、秋季养生（Regimen in Autumn）

秋季从立秋之日起,至立冬之日止,包括立秋、处暑、白露、秋分、寒露、霜降 6 个节气。《素问·四气调神大论》:"秋三月,此谓容平。天气以急,地气以明。"秋天气候由热转寒,较为干燥,万物成熟而平定收藏,阳气渐退,阴气渐长,是万物成熟收获的季节。秋应五脏之肺,属金。秋凉秋收,人体阳气也开始内敛,阴气渐生。因此,秋季养生凡精神情志、饮食起居、运动锻炼皆以养收为原则,保持阴阳平衡,注意秋冬养阴,防止燥邪伤肺。

秋季应早睡早起,以顺应秋季自然界阳气由疏泄趋向收敛的变化特点。在衣着方面,天气渐凉,应注意根据天气适当添加衣被。随着天气逐渐干燥,皮肤干燥的人群,易出现皮肤脱屑、瘙痒的情况,因此日常洗浴不宜过于频繁,不宜过热,沐浴后应涂抹保湿剂;秋季应安心静养、情绪慢慢收敛,保持安宁平静,凡事不躁进亢奋,不畏缩郁结,使肺气清肃才能适应自然界"秋气平"的特点,符合秋季养"收"的养生要求,日常可外出秋游、登高远眺、赏菊花、观红叶等保持心胸豁达、情绪乐观;饮食方面,可常备生姜、大葱、紫苏等具有一定发散作用的食物。秋季是开展各项运动锻炼的大好时期,如跑步、跳绳、拔河、打拳、练功等运动时,要在空气清新和避风的地方,防止运动过量出现劳累大汗的情况,运动后注意不要汗出当风。

四、冬季养生（Regimen in Winter）

冬季从立冬之日起,至立春之日止,包括立冬、小雪、大雪、冬至、小寒、大寒 6 个节气,是一年中气候最冷的季节。《素问·四气调神大论》曰:"冬三月,此谓闭藏。水冰地坼,无扰乎阳。"冬季天寒地冻,大地龟裂,北风凛冽,草木凋零,蛰虫伏藏,生机潜伏,阳气内藏,是万物闭藏的季节。冬应五脏之肾,五行属水,此季节寒冷,与人体的肾和膀胱关系密切。冬寒冬藏,从生理角度讲,人体在夏季阳气潜藏于内,新陈代谢较慢,阴阳消长也处于相对缓慢的水平,成形胜于化气。因此,冬季养生基本原则为"藏",在藏精养阴的同时,也要回避虚邪贼风。

为了适应冬季日照减少、万物封藏的自然规律,在起居方面应注意调整,日出后起床,保证足够睡眠,不应当扰动阳气。日出而作,日落而息,以利阳气潜藏,阴精积蓄。在衣着方面,冬季穿衣应本着"去寒就温"的养藏原则,防寒保暖,不仅衣料选择要注意保暖,帽子、围巾、手套也都应配套。冬季人体容易出现精神抑郁、情绪低沉等情况,需进行自我主观调节,如听欢快的音乐、与友人畅谈、读书、运动等,都有利于摆脱低落情绪;冬季天寒地冻,阳气闭藏,人体处于能量蓄积状态,需要比夏季更多的热量来御寒,适合吃温性食物如大枣、果仁、龙眼肉、羊肉、牛肉、鹿肉等做适当进补;冬季不宜进行剧烈运动,避免汗出过多,防止风寒冰霜所伤,运动前要注意做好热身,防止运动损伤。

People live between heaven and earth. As there is correspondence between man and nature, following the laws of climate change in nature helps people keep healthy. If the climate change in nature goes against the routine, bringing about abnormal occurrence, people will be affected to a certain extent under the influence of correspondence. According to *Shanghan Lun* (*Treatise on Febrile Diseases*), "It is warm in spring, hot in summer, cool in autumn and cold in winter. This is the normal climate change law". This is the law of normal climate change in nature. Under this law, diseases will reflect, to a certain extent, the characteristics of normal climate change accordingly. For example, as is stated in *Jinkui Zhenyan Lun* of *Su Wen* (*Discussion on Important Ideas in the Golden Chamber*, the chapter of *Plain Conversation*), "that is why *Qiunü* (nasal stuffiness and bleeding) is usually seen in spring; chest and rib-side disorders are often seen in summer; *Hanzhong* (internal cold syndromes) like *Dongxie* (acute diarrhea) are frequently seen in late summer; *Fengnue* (Wind-Malaria) is often seen in autumn and *Bijue* (numbness and coldness of the four limbs) is always seen in winter." It is also recorded in *Shanghan Lun* that "*Shixing* refers to abnormal seasonal climate when it is cold in spring, cool in summer, hot in autumn and warm in winter. At that time, men and women, old and young, will suffer from similar diseases due to the invasion of evil *qi*." It shows that the similar diseases are caused by abnormal climate changes.

1 Regimen in Spring

Spring starts from *Lichun* (Beginning of Spring) and ends in *Lixia* (Beginning of Summer), including six solar terms that are *Lichun* (Beginning of Spring), *Yushui* (Rain Water), *Jingzhe* (Awakening of Insects), *Chunfen* (Spring Equinox), *Qingming* (Clear and Bright) and *Guyu* (Grain Rain). Spring is the first of the four seasons, and Beginning of Spring is the first solar term. It is said in *Siqi Tiaoshen Dalun* of *Su Wen* (*Major Discussion of Regulation of Spirit According to the Changes of the Four Seasons*, the chapter of *Plain* (*conversation*) that "all things on the earth begin to grow in the three months of spring. The natural world is resuscitating and all things are flourishing", which describes the scene that natural world is full of vitality and prosperity when spring returns to the earth and *yang qi* rises. Spring pertains to the liver of the five *zang*-organs, and the wood of Five-Elements, and it is also a time when the liver *qi* is smooth. Physiologically, as spring is warm and everything grows, it will raise *yang qi* in human body. People should conform to the rule that *yang* rises in spring and everything begins to grow when in eating, living, exercising and thinking, maintaining the rising *qi*.

In the health preservation in spring, we should pay attention to the rising of *yang qi* and the smoothness of liver *qi*. In daily life, it is better to sleep at night and get up in the morning, be bareheaded and let hair down, and wear loose clothes so as to stretch the *qi* movement and body. In terms of clothing, even if the weather turns warm, it is not suggested to take off clothes quickly, especially for the elderly and the infirm and people with basic diseases. Be careful not to take off thick clothes suddenly. That's because the temperature is not stable in seasonal transition, so clothing alteration should not be too much or too soon. In spring, attention should be paid to the recurrence of mental disorders. Various ways can be adopted to keep an open and happy mind, such as going for an outing and chanting, which can help people relax and develop a moderated and optimistic mentality by cultivating temperament and refreshing body and mind. In spring, it is advisable to eat food in pungent and sweet taste, such as leeks, green onions, onions, ginger. Instead of those in sour taste, which helps to nourish and raise *yang*. As it gradually warms up in spring, people wear less clothes accordingly, which eases the burden of the body. Going to somewhere with fresh air, climbing mountains and appreciating flowers are all good choices for health preservation by exercising in spring, but too much exercise leads to exhaustion. Check whether clothes and shoes are suitable before exercise. Wear shoes and socks that are elastic and moisture–wicking. For patients with cardiovascular and cerebrovascular diseases, choose the right exercise and do what you can.

2 Regimen in Summer

Summer, a season with the most *yang qi*, starts from *Lixia* (Start of Summer) and ends in *Liqiu* (Start of Autumn), including six solar terms: *Lixia* (Start of Summer), *Xiaoman* (Grain Buds), *Mangzhong* (Grain in Ear), *Xiazhi* (Summer Solstice), *Xiaoshu* (Minor Heat) and *Dashu* (Major Heat). It is said in *Siqi Tiaoshen Dalun* of *Su Wen* (*Major Discussion of Regulation of Spirit According to the Changes of the Four Seasons*, the chapterof *Plain* (*conversation*) that "The three months of summer is the period of prosperity. *Tianqi* (Heaven–*qi*) and *Diqi* (Earth–*qi*) have converged and all things are in blossom". In summer, everything is luxuriant and beautiful, and *yang qi* is exuberant. It is a season when everything grows and matures and a period when utmost *yang* brings about *yin*. Summer pertains to the heart and the fire. Summer is hot and long. Physiologically, *yang qi* is also exuberant exteriorly. Health preservation in summer should observe the law, focusing on the maintenance and increment of *yang*. To nourish the five *zang*–organs, heart is prioritized. In addition, as the long summer is wet and rainy, there is damp heat transpiration between heaven and earth, which corresponds to the spleen.

However, the spleen has preference to dryness and aversion to dampness, so it is easy to get hurt at this time. Therefore, it is suggested to invigorate the spleen in health preservation in long summer.

In the hot summer, we should reduce strenuous activities during the day, and go to cooler places. Wear sun hats, sunglasses and use parasols when going out. As it is easy to sweat often in midsummer, take bath and change clothes frequently to keep skin and dress clean. One may feel impetuous due to the hot weather. But it can be improved by maintaining a peaceful and pleased mind. Listening to soothing music, drinking green tea and practicing calligraphy are also helpful. Besides, as the pathogenic cold will easily invade the lung, it is advised to eat pungent foods such as radish, scallion, ginger and garlic, leek moss, but do not eat too much. Sweating is more often in summer due to the opening striae and interstices, so it is recommended to eat some sour food, which helps to converge the striae and interstices as well as generate fluid to quench thirst, such as sour plum soup. Avoid exercising in the heat, especially at noon with the strongest sunshine and highest temperature, to prevent heatstroke. It is best to exercise in the cooler parts of the day such as morning and evening, and in places with fresh air like parks, courtyards and shoreline. Avoid strenuous exercise to prevent the consumption of *qi* and fluid caused by excessive sweat. Exercises like Swimming, walking, jogging, Taichi and calisthenics are more appropriate. Replenish water during exercise, and don't take a cold shower immediately after exercise.

3   Regimen in Autumn

Autumn starts from *Liqiu* (Start of Autumn) and ends in *Lidong* (Start of Winter), including six solar terms: Start of Autumn, *Chushu* (End of Heat), *Bailu* (White Dew), *Qiufen* (Autumn Equinox), *Hanlu* (Cold Dew), *Shuangjiang* (Frost's Descent). It is said in *Siqi Tiaoshen Dalun* of *Su Wen* (*Major Discussion of Regulation of Spirit According to the Changes of the Four Seasons*, the chapter of *Plain Conversation*) that "The three months of autumn is the season of *Rongping* (ripening). In autumn it is cool, the wind blows fast and the atmosphere is clear". Autumn, changing from hot to cold, is relatively dry. All things mature. It is a harvest season when *yang* is gradually fading and *yin* is growing. And autumn pertains to the lung and the metal. *Yang qi* begins to go inward and astringe while *yin qi* starts to grow in the cool season. Therefore, eating, living, exercising and thinking in autumn should be based on the principle of not consuming too much *yang qi*, keeping the balance between *yin* and *yang*, and nourishing *yin* in autumn and winter to prevent pathogenic dryness from hurting the lung.

Also, we should go to bed early and get up early, conforming to the characteristics of *yang qi* in autumn. In terms of clothing, add clothes and quilts properly as it is getting colder. When the weather gradually dries up, people with dry skin are prone to desquamation and itching, so do not take a frequent or overheated shower and apply humectant to skin after bathing. Have a good rest and keep a peaceful mind. Do not cringe or overexcite. In this way, the lung–*qi* can be clear, and *yin* and *yang* in balance. Autumn outing, climbing, and the appreciation of chrys-anthemum and red leaves are advisable to keep open – minded and optimistic. In terms of diet, recommended food are ginger, green onions, perilla that have dispersing effect. Autumn is a great time for exercises such as running, skipping, tug-of-war, boxing, and *gong*-practicing. Choose a place with fresh air and without wind. Avoid too much exercise to prevent excessive fatigue and sweat. Be careful not to be invaded by pathogenic wind after sweating.

4 Regimen in Winter

Winter, the coldest season in the whole year, starts from Start of Winter and ends in Start of Spring, including six solar terms: Start of Winter, *Xiaoxue* (Minor Snow), *Daxue* (Major Snow), *Dongzhi* (Winter Solstice), *Xiaohan* (Minor Cold) and *Dahan* (Major Cold). It is said in *Siqi Tiaoshen Dalun* of *Su Wen* (*Major Discussion of Regulation of Spirit According to the Changes of the Four Seasons*, the chapter of *Plain Conversation*) that "The three months of winter is the season for storage. The water freezes and the earth cracks. Cares must be taken not to disturb *yang*." In cold winter, there is cracked earth, biting north wind, withered vegetation, hidden insects. It is a season for storage as vitality is lurking and *yang* is hidden. Winter pertains to the kidney and the water. And this cold season is closely related to kidney and bladder. Physiologically, *yang qi* is hidden in the human body and metabolism is slow. The waning and waxing of *yin* and *yang* is also slow, and it is better to form shape than transform to *qi*. Therefore, the basic principle of preserving health in winter is to promote the storing function of the body. While hiding essence and nourishing *yin*, people should also avoid deficiency–evil and thief wind.

In order to adapt to the natural law that sunshine hours are reduced and all creature store energy in winter, it is suggested to get up after sunrise, which ensures enough sleep. And *yang qi* should not be disturbed. Go to work when the sun rises, and come back to rest when the sun sets, which facilitates the hiding of *yang qi* and the accumulation of *yin* and essence. Dressing in winter should be based on the principle of "preventing cold and keeping warm". Not only should people choose warm clothing, but also wear hats, scarves and gloves. It is easy to be in a low mood in winter, so self-adjustment is necessary such as listening to cheerful music, talking with friends, reading, exercising, which is conducive to getting rid of depression.

Furthermore, human body is in a state of storing energy, which requires more heat to keep out the cold than in summer. It is advisable to eat warm – natured food such as jujube, nuts, longan meat, mutton, beef and venison. Strenuous exercise is not advisable because excessive sweating will make body vulnerable to wind cold and frost. Warm-up before exercise is important to prevent sports injuries.

第三节　食物的四性与五味
（Four Properties and Five Flavors of Food）

一、食物的四性（Four Properties of Food）

食物的性能古称"食性""食气""食味"等,是古人在长期生活与临床实践中对食物的保健和医疗作用的经验总结。选择食物必须"于人脏腑有宜",因此,需要运用中医药理论中的四气、五味、升降浮沉以及药物归经等学说来分析食物的作用。现代研究表明,各种食物所含成分及其含量多少均不同,因此对人体的保健作用也不同,从而表现出各自性能。食物的性能主要包括四气、五味、升降浮沉、归经等。历代中医食疗书籍所载的食性很多,如大热、热、大温、温、微温、平、凉、微寒、大寒等,中医称为"四性"或"四气",即指食物所具有的寒、热、温、凉四种不同的性质,其中温热与寒凉属于两类不同的性质。热与温、寒与凉有其共性,但程度上有所不同,温次于热,凉次于寒。还有一类食物寒热性质都不太明显,作用比较和缓,则归于平性。因此,可以把食物分为寒凉、温热、平性三类。

确定食物的"性",是从食物作用于机体所发生的反应中概括而出,与食物的食用效果一致。寒、凉性质的食物,如西瓜、绿豆、萝卜、茄子、紫菜、螃蟹等,具有清热泻火、凉血解毒、平肝安神、通利二便等作用,适用于热性病证,临床表现为发热、面红目赤、口渴心烦、小便黄赤、舌苔黄燥、大便秘结、脉数或沉实有力等,此类食物是阳热亢盛、肝火偏旺者首选的保健膳食。热、温性质的食物,如羊肉、黄牛肉、狗肉、姜、辣椒等,具有温中散寒、助阳益气、通经活血等作用,适用于寒性病证,临床表现为喜暖怕冷、手脚冰冷、口不渴、小便清长、大便稀薄等,此类食物是冬季御寒的保健食品。常用食物四性归类如下:①寒性食物,如龙须菜、海带、茼蒿、马齿苋、苦菜、梨子、苦瓜等;②凉性食物,如茄子、丝瓜、莴苣、绿豆、橙子、枇杷、橄榄等;③热性食物,如胡椒、芥末、肉桂、干姜、辣椒等;④温性食物,如荔枝、洋葱、糯米、胡桃仁、鳝鱼等。

二、食物的五味（Five Flavors of Food）

食物的味概括为辛、甘、酸、苦、咸五味。除五味之外,还有"淡"味和"涩"味,长期以来将"淡附于甘""涩附于酸"，以合五行配属关系，所以习称"五味"。辛，实际上包括麻、辣等刺激性滋味和清香气（本草多称辛香）；甘，除表示味甜外，也指一些食性平和、可食而近于淡味者；酸，有时也包括近于酸的涩味；只有苦、咸是单一的味。《食疗本草》中对食物确定的味大多数与其实际滋味相符，但随着实践发展，古人不再只用尝试的办法来定味，而主要由其功能来推定。如已知咸味有软坚散结等作用，若某种食物有这种作用即可定为咸味，如石莼、昆布、蛤蜊；具有滋养补益作用的肉类、内脏定为甘味，实际并无甜味。《黄帝内经》指出："天食人以五气，地食人以五味……五味入口，藏于肠胃，味有所藏，以养五气，气和而生，津液相成，神乃自生。"认为人体五脏之气，气血津液的生成，神气的健旺，完全依赖于天地间五气、五味的供养，而五味的来源就是自然界的各种食物。食物的五味不同，其功效各异。

1. 辛味　辛味散行，有发散、行气、活血、通窍、化湿等作用，主治外感表证、气滞、血瘀、窍闭、湿阻等。如风寒感冒者，可选用生姜、葱白、大蒜等辛味的食材，以宣散风寒；痹证患者，可选用白酒或药酒，以散寒祛湿，温经活血。此外，辛味还有调味、健胃的效用，如寒凝气滞引起的胃痛患者可选用辣椒、砂仁、茴香等，以行气、散寒、止痛；同时，辛味食物多兼有香味或辣味，是餐桌上必不可少的调味品。常用的辛味食材有葱、生姜、蒜、芥菜、薤白、酒、花椒、胡椒、辣椒、桂皮等。

2. 甘（淡）味　甘味能补、能和、能缓，有补益、调和、缓急止痛等作用，主治虚证（或营养不良）、脾胃不和、拘急腹痛等。如脾胃气虚及胃阳不足诸证，可选用糯米、红枣等甘味食材，以补气、温中；气滞拘急的腹痛，可选饴糖、甘草缓急止痛。甘味又有较好的调味、矫味的作用，如白糖、红糖、蜂蜜、甜叶菊等。常用的甘味食材有山药、南瓜、银耳、鸡肉、龙眼肉、甜杏仁、荔枝、大枣、饴糖、甘草以乃各种动物的肉。

3. 酸（涩）味　酸味收涩，有开胃、生津、收敛、固涩等作用，主治体虚虚汗、肺虚久咳、久泻脱、遗精遗尿、崩漏带下等。如气虚卫外不固所致的多汗，可选用梅子、刺梨、五味子等止汗；泄泻、尿频、遗精、滑精诸症，可摄取莲子、芡实等酸味食物。其次，酸味食物又有生津止渴或消食的功能。常用的酸味食材有梅子、酸角、柠檬、醋柳果、刺梨、山楂、醋等。

4. 苦味　苦味泄燥，有清热、泻火、燥湿等作用，主治湿热、实火等。如夏天热郁成痱时，多用苦瓜、西瓜清热解暑；热证的便秘心烦，可选用莲子、莴苣等清热除烦。常用的苦味食材有苦瓜、莴笋叶、青果、芥菜、枸杞苗、罗布麻、茶叶等。但是过食苦味易导致消化不良，尤其是骨病患者不宜多食。

5. 咸味　咸味软下，有泻下通便、软坚散结等作用，主治大便秘结、瘰疬瘿瘤、痰核、痞块等。如瘰疬、痰核、痞块，可选用海带、昆布等软坚散结；大便燥结，可选用海蜇、淡盐水润肠通便。淡鸭肉补肾，乌贼、猪蹄补血养阴。常用的咸味食材有昆布、紫菜、海藻、蛤蜊、海蜇、海参等。

在进食时，味不可偏亢。偏亢太过容易伤及五脏，对健康不利。过多食用咸味食物会瘀滞血脉,过多食用苦味食物可使皮肤枯槁、毛发脱落,过多食用辛味食物会引起筋脉拘挛、爪甲干枯不荣,过多食用酸味食物会使肌肉失去光泽、变粗变硬甚至口唇翻起,过多食用甜味食品则会使骨骼疼痛、头发脱落。由于每种食物都具有性和味,因此两者必须结合起来看,如两种食物都是寒(凉)性,但一是苦寒(凉),一是辛凉,性虽相同而味不同,两者的作用就存在差异,前者能清热泻火,后者可发散风热。因此,不能把性与味孤立。

1　Four Properties of Food

The performance of food, also called food nature, food *qi* and food taste in ancient times, is a summary of the ancient people's experience on the health-care and medical effect of food in their long life and clinical practice. People should choose food that is beneficial to viscera. Therefore, it is necessary to analyze the role of food by using the theories of four properties, five flavors, ascending, descending, floating and sinking as well as meridian tropism in TCM. Modern research shows that various foods differ in component types and content, so they have different health-care effects on human body, thus showing their own performances. The performance of food mainly includes four properties, five flavors, ascending, descending, floating and sinking, meridian tropism. Food properties have been recorded in Chinese medicine dietotherapy books in the past, such as greatly heat, heat, greatly warm, warm, slightly warm, neutral, cool, slightly cold, greatly cold. In TCM, they are also known as "four properties" or "four *qi*", which mainly refer to cold, hot, warm and cool. They can be classified into two types: one is warm and hot; the other is cold and cool. Hot and warm have their commonalities, so do cold and cool. But they represent varying degrees of heat and cold. There is also a kind of food whose property is not obvious and has mild effect, which can be attributed to neutral. Hence, food can be classified into three categories: cold and cool, warm and hot as well as neutral.

The property of food is determined by summarizing the body reaction after taking food, which is consistent with the eating effect. Food in cold and cool nature, such as watermelon, mung bean, radish, eggplant, laver, crab, have the effect of clearing heat and purging fire, cooling blood and detoxifying, calming liver and tranquilizing mind, and promoting urination and defecation. They are indicated to heat syndromes manifested as fever, flushed cheeks and red eyes, thirst and upset, dark urine, yellow and dry tongue coating, constipation, as well as deep and rapid pulse. These are the first choice for people with exuberant *yang*-heat and liver-fire. Food in cold and cool nature, such as mutton, beef, dog meat, ginger, pepper, have the effect of warming the middle-*jiao* and dispelling cold, invigorating *yang* and supplementing *qi*, dredging collaterals and promoting blood circulation. They are indicated to cold syndromes manifested as preference to warm and aversion to cold, cold hands and feet, no thirsty, clear and abundant urine, loose stool, etc. These are health food for keeping out the cold in winter. Common food classified by four properties: ①Cold-natured food: *Longxu cai* (*Asparagus schoberioides Kunth*), kelp, crowndaisy chrysanthemum, purslane, bitter herb, pear, bitter gourd, etc.; ②Cool-natured food: eggplant, towel gourd, lettuce, mung bean, orange, loquat, olive, etc.; ③Hot-natured food: pepper, mustard, cinnamon, dried ginger, pepper, etc.; ④Warm-natured food: litchi, onion, glutinous rice, walnut kernel, eel, etc.

2　Five Flavors of Food

Five flavors refer to pungent, sweet, sour, bitter and salty. Additionally, there are also bland and astringent. For a long time, bland is attributed to sweet and astringent to sour so as to attach to the Five-Elements, so they are often called five flavors. Pungent actually includes intense tastes such as acrid and spicy, and aroma (referring to that of herbs). Sweet, in addition to the sweet taste, also contains a bland taste. Sour, sometimes includes astringent. Only bitter and salty refer to a single taste. Most of the flavors are determined by the actual taste of food in *Shiliao Bencao* (*Materia Medica for Dietotherapy*). However, with the development of practice, the ancients no longer determined the flavors by singly tasting, but made presumption by their functions. For example, salty is known to have the function of softening and dissolving, so the food with this function can be said to have a salty taste, such as *shichun* (*Ulva lactuca Linnaeus*), kelp and clam. Also, the meat and internal organs having the function of nourishing and tonifying are considered to have a sweet taste, but they do not taste sweet in fact. It is stated in *Huangdi Neijing* that "The heavens provide man with five kinds of *qi* and the earth provides man with five kinds of flavors. When the five kinds of flavors are taken in through the mouth and stored in the intestines and the stomach, their nutrients infuse into the five *zang*-organs to nourish the five kinds of *qi*. The harmony of *qi* (visceral-*qi*) ensures the production of the *Jinye* (body fluid) and *Shen* (spirit)." It is believed that the generation of visceral-*qi*, blood and body fluid as well as sufficient spirit are entirely supported by the five *qi* and five flavors between heaven and earth, and the latter come from various food in nature. And the food with different flavors varies in function.

2.1　Pungent

It has the functions of dispersing, promoting *qi* and blood circulation, opening orifices, removing dampness, etc. It is indicated for exterior syndromes, *qi* stagnation, blood stasis, orifice closure, dampness obstruction, etc. For example, patients with a wind-cold can eat pungent food such as ginger,scallion and garlic to dispel the wind-cold pathogens. And patients with arthralgia syndrome can drink Chinese Baijiu or medicinal wine to dissipate cold and dampness,warm meridians and promote blood circulation. In addition,pungent has the effect of seasoning and invigorating stomach. For example, pepper, *sharen* (*Amomum villosum Lour.*),fennel can be used by patients with stomachache caused by cold coagulation and *qi* stagnation to promote *qi* circulation,dispel cold and relieve pain. Meanwhile, pungent food is mostly spicy,which is an essential condiment on the table. Common food includes onion,ginger,garlic,mustard, *xiebai* (*Allium macrostemon Bunge*) , wine,pepper,cinnamon and so on.

2.2 Sweet (balnd)

Sweet taste can tonify, harmonize and moderate, which can also be used to relieve pain,etc. It is indicated for deficiency syndrome (or malnutrition),disharmony between spleen and stomach,acute abdominal pain,etc. For example,sweet food such as glutinous rice and red dates can be used to relieve the syndromes of *qi* deficiency of spleen and stomach as well as *yang* deficiency of stomach by invigorating *qi* and warming the middle *jiao*. For abdominal pain caused by *qi* stagnation,maltose and licorice can be used to relieve it. Sweet taste has an effect of seasoning,including white sugar,brown sugar,honey,stevia and so on. Common sweet food includes yam,pumpkin,tremella,chicken,longan,sweet almond,litchi,jujube,maltose and licorice as well as the meat of various animals.

2.3 Sour (astringent)

Sour has the functions of appetizing, promoting fluid production, absorbing and controlling,etc. It is indicated to deficiency syndromes such as abnormal sweating due to debility,chronic cough due to lung deficiency,chronic diarrhea and anal prolapse,spermatorrhea and enuresis,metrorrhagia and leukorrhagia. For hyperhidrosis caused by *qi* deficiency failing to protect against exogenous pathogens, plum, *cili* (*Rosa roxburghii*) and *wuwei zi* (*Schisandra chinensis*) can be used to stop sweating. For diarrhea,frequent urination,spermatorrhea and so on,lotus seeds and gorgon fruit can be taken to relieve syndromes. Also,sour food can produce body fluid to quench thirst or promote digestion. Common sour food includes plum,tamarind,lemon,sea buckthorn, *cili* (*Rosa roxburghii*) ,hawthorn,vinegar and so on.

2.4 Bitter

Bitter has the functions of drying,clearing heat,purging fire,etc. ,and is indicated for syndromes of damp heat and excess fire. For example,when miliaria occurs in summer,bitter gourd and watermelon can be used to beat summer heat. Lotus seeds and lettuce can be used to treat heat syndrome manifested as constipation and vexation by clearing heat and relieving restlessness. Commonly used bitter food includes melon, lettuce leaves, Chinese olive, leaf mustard, Chinese wolfberry leaf, dogbane, tea and so on. However, overeating bitter food can easily lead to indigestion, especially for patients with osteopathy.

2.5　Salty

Salty has the functions of purging, promoting defecation, softening hardness and releasing hardening and nodules. It is indicated for syndromes such as constipation, scrofula, goiter and tumor, subcutaneous nodule and abdominal lump. For scrofula, subcutaneous nodule and abdominal lump, kelp can be used to soften and dissolve. For dry bound stool, jellyfish and light salt water can be used to relax bowels. Unsalted duck meat is used to tonify kidney, squid and pig's trotters to replenishing blood and nourish *yin*. Commonly used salty food includes kelp, laver, seaweed, clam, jellyfish, sea cucumber and so on.

It is not suggested to eat food with strong flavors, because it is likely to damage five *zang*-organs, which does harm to health. Overeating of salty food will cause blood stasis. Over intake of bitter food will lead to duller skin and hair shedding. Overeating of pungent food will result in tendon spasm and dry nail. Eating too much sour food will make the muscles thicken, harden and less lustrous, and even the lips will turn up. And too much sweet food will cause bone pain and hair loss. Every food has its property and flavor, which must be put together. For example, there are two kinds of food that both are in cold (cool) nature, but one is bitter in taste, the other is pungent. Despite the shared nature, they have different functions due to different tastes. The former can clear away heat and purge fire, while the latter can dispel wind-heat. Therefore, the properties and flavors of food cannot be separated.

第四节　药食同源
（Food and Medicine Coming from the Same Source）

对于"药食同源"目前尚无统一的定义,药食同源是我国人民在生产实践中认识药物和食物并对两者关系的概括,即药物与食物具有同源性,具体指药物和食物都来源于自然界,都以初生代谢产物和次生化代谢产物为物质基础,在中医药理论指导下应用于实践。药物和食物中代谢产物类型及比例的差异使得两者的性味及功效有差异,进而使得食物侧重于养生,药物多用于治病。

一、药食同源与药食两用物质的定义（Definition）

药食同源是人们对食物和药物（尤其是中药材）关系的归纳,指食物与药物来源一致,且具有成分同源性和理论同源性,许多食物既有食用性又有药用性,因此可用以养生保健及防病治病。药食同源是一种观念,不指代具体的物质。

药食两用物质是对药食同源更具体、更科学的阐释。在广义上,凡是既可食用又可药用的物质皆为药食两用物质。从《食疗本草》的 260 种药食两用物质到《食物本草》的1679 种,古代医家们对药食两用物质的范围不断扩充。而后,在安全可控原则的指导下,在对药食两用物质成分及长期服用的安全性充分研究的基础上,从古代食物类本草中规范筛选安全性好的 87 种到《既是食品又是药品的物品名单》,经修订逐渐规范了药食两用物质的品种,进而明确了"按照传统既是食品又是中药材物质"(药食同源物/药食两用物质)的定义、列入原则、来源、使用部位和限制使用等信息,为药食两用物质的应用提供了科学的指导。药食两用物质是具有传统食用习惯,且列入国家中药材标准(《中华人民共和国药典》及相关中药材标准)中的动物和植物可使用部分(食品原料、香辛料和调味品)。

二、药食同源的内涵(Connotation)

(一)来源具有同源性

食物和药物均来源于自然界,人类对于食物的认识早于药物,在觅食的过程中,人们逐渐认识到某些物质能填饱肚子,即将其确定为食物;某些物质能损人健康或致人死亡,即为毒物;某些物质能使患病之人好转,即为药物。在我国,食物和药物的发现往往归功于神农氏。《医膳》中解释神农尝百草是"为别民之可食者,而非定医药也",也说明寻食先于定药,即药食本同源,然先寻食后得药。以植物为主的饮食习惯,加上药物又多从植物而来,我国的药物亦称为"本草",可视为药食同源的例证。随着人类实践活动发展和认识水平的提高,人们认识到食物和药物的不同特性而将两者分离开来,药与食由同源走向分化,同时衍生了药食两用的分支。

(二)成分具有同源性

从生物和化学的角度说,组成生命的元素相同,均为碳、氢、氧、氮、硫、磷等,这些基本元素进一步构成蛋白质、脂肪、氨基酸和糖类等初生代谢产物,初生代谢产物通过次生代谢过程产生萜类、黄酮类、酚类和生物碱类等次生代谢产物。就功能而言,初生代谢产物可满足人体对能量的需求,而次生代谢产物多为防治疾病的有效成分。自 20 世纪 60年代日本提出"功能食品"的概念以来,世界各国纷纷投入食品的功能性成分研究中。膳食纤维、类胡萝卜素、低聚果糖等被认为是有益健康的功能性成分。因此,食品除营养功能和感官功能外,还衍生了第三功能,即保健功能。此外,学者们将目光投向食物和药物的共有成分,并重点研究这些共有成分的保健功效及其机制。如葡萄、桑椹和虎杖中的白藜芦醇,具有抗肿瘤、抗心血管疾病、抗炎、抑菌抗病毒、免疫调节和雌激素样作用(可缓解更年期综合征）。如多糖,广泛存在于食物和药物中,具有修复肠道屏障及调节肠道微生态、抗氧化、降血糖、降血脂、提高免疫等药理作用。因此,食物和药物在成分上的同源性,为两者应用于医疗保健奠定了物质基础。

（三）理论具有同源性

由于药物和食物来源相同,且共同目标是使人健康,客观上要求两者须有共同的理论指导。我国药食同源理念在应用于实践时体现了鲜明的中医药特色,食物和药物的理论同源性,主要体现在整体观念和辨证论治思想指导下的药食运用法则上。整体观、平衡观、阴阳五行、性味归经、升降浮沉、三因制宜等理论指导着食物和药物的应用。

三、药食同源物品（Items）

卫生部于 2002 年发布的《卫生部关于进一步规范保健食品原料管理的通知》（卫法监发〔2002〕51 号）中,列出既是食品又是药品的物品有 86 个,分别有丁香、八角茴香、刀豆、小茴香、小蓟、山药、山楂、马齿苋、乌梢蛇、乌梅、木瓜、火麻仁、代代花、玉竹、甘草、白芷、白果、白扁豆、白扁豆花、龙眼肉（桂圆）、决明子、百合、肉豆蔻、肉桂、余甘子、佛手、杏仁（甜、苦）、沙棘、牡蛎、芡实、花椒、赤小豆、阿胶、鸡内金、麦芽、昆布、枣（大枣、酸枣、黑枣）、罗汉果、郁李仁、金银花、青果、鱼腥草、姜（生姜、干姜）、枳椇子、枸杞子、栀子、砂仁、胖大海、茯苓、香橼、香薷、桃仁、桑叶、桑椹、橘红、桔梗、益智仁、荷叶、莱菔子、莲子、高良姜、淡竹叶、淡豆豉、菊花、菊苣、黄芥子、黄精、紫苏、紫苏籽、葛根、黑芝麻、黑胡椒、槐米、槐花、蒲公英、蜂蜜、榧子、酸枣仁、鲜白茅根、鲜芦根、蝮蛇、橘皮、薄荷、薏苡仁、薤白、覆盆子、藿香。

国家卫生计划生育委员会于 2014 年 11 月发布《按照传统既是食品又是中药材物质目录管理办法》征求意见稿,在之前被列入《既是食品又是药品的物品名单》的 86 种药食同源目录基础上,新增人参、山银花、芫荽、玫瑰花、松花粉（马尾松和油松）、粉葛、布渣叶、夏枯草、当归、山奈、西红花、草果、姜黄、荜茇 15 种药食同源品种。

2019 年 11 月,国家卫生健康委员会、国家市场监管总局联合印发《关于对党参等 9 种物质开展按照传统既是食品又是中药材的物质管理试点工作的通知》（国卫食品函〔2019〕311 号）,提出将对党参、肉苁蓉、铁皮石斛、西洋参、黄芪、灵芝、山茱萸、天麻、杜仲叶 9 种物质开展按照传统既是食品又是中药材的物质的生产经营试点工作。

At present, there is no unified definition of "*Yaoshi Tongyuan*". It refers to people's understanding of medicine and food as well as their relationship acquired in practice, that is, medicine and food have shared source. More specifically, it means that both medicine and food come from nature, which is based on primary metabolites and secondary biochemical metabolites, and is put into practice under the guidance of TCM theory. The difference in the types and proportions of metabolites between medicine and food makes them different in property, flavor and efficacy. That's why food is mostly used for health preservation and medicine for treating diseases.

1　Definition

Yaoshi Tongyuan indicates the relationship between food and medicine (especially Chinese herbal medicines), which means that food and medicine have the same source, and there is homology of component and theory between them. Many foods are both edible and medicinal, so they can be used for health care and disease prevention and treatment. It is a concept, not referring to specific substances.

And *Yaoshi liangyong* gives a more specific and scientific explanation. In a broad sense, it refers to all edible and medicinal substance. It can be seen that ancient physicians have continuously expanded the scope of medicinal and edible substance, as the recorded number of edible and medicinal substance has increased to 1679 in *Shiliao Bencao* (*Materia Medica for Dietotherapy*) from 260 in *Shiwu Bencao* (*Materia Medica Food*). Then, guided by the principle of safety and controllability and based on the study of the components and safety for long−term use, 87 kinds were added to the *List of Varieties that Are Both Food and Medicine* after being screened from ancient food herbs. The varieties of medicinal and edible substances were gradually standardized after revision. Moreover, it clarified the definition, inclusion principle, source, used part and restriction of medicinal and edible substances, which provides scientific guidance for the application of medicinal and edible substances. Medicinal and edible substances are the usable parts of animals and plants (food raw materials, spices and condiments) with traditional eating habits and listed in the national Chinese herbal medicine standards (*Pharmacopoeia of the People's Republic of China* and related standards).

2　Connotation

2.1　Shared Origin

Both food and medicine come from nature, but human beings know food earlier than medicine. When searching for food, people gradually realize that some substances can satisfy their hunger, so they call these substances food. Substances that do harm to people's health or cause death are considered as poisons. Substances that can treat diseases are known as medicine. In China, it was *Shennong* who discovered food and medicine. It is explained in *Yi Sheng*(a medical history book compiled by Danbo Yuanjian in 1788) that *Shennong* tasted hundreds of herbs "with the purpose of finding food for people, rather than medicine", which also shows that people searched for food first and then medicine. It can also be said that medicine and food come from the same source. Because of the plant-based diet and the fact that many medicines come from plants, Chinese medicines are also called "materia medica", which can be regarded as evidence of the concept that medicine and food come from the same source. With the development of human activities and the improvement of cognitive level, people realize and separate the different characteristics of food and medicine. Therefore, medicine and food are differentiated, and a branch of edible medicinal substance is derived at the same time.

2.2 Shared Source in Components

Biologically and chemically, all living things have basic elements in common, which are carbon, hydrogen, oxygen, nitrogen, sulfur, phosphorus, etc. These elements constitute primary metabolites such as protein, fat, amino acid and carbohydrate, which will produce secondary metabolites such as terpenes, flavonoids, phenols and alkaloids through secondary metabolism. In terms of function, primary metabolites can provide energy that humans require, while secondary metabolites are mostly effective components for prevention and treatment of diseases. Since the concept of "functional food" was put forward by Japan in 1960s, countries from all over the world have devoted themselves to the research of functional components of food. Dietary fiber, carotenoids and fructooligosaccharides are considered as functional components beneficial to health. Therefore, food can also provide health benefits except for nutrient and sensory properties. In addition, the researchers focus on the shared components of food and medicine, especially their health care effects and mechanisms. For example, resveratrol in grapes, mulberry and polygonum cuspidatum has effects of anti-tumor, anti-cardiovascular disease, anti-inflammation, anti-bacterial and anti-virus. It also has ennancing regulation and estrogen-like effect. For another example, polysaccharide, which exists in most of food and medicine, has pharmacological effects including repairing intestinal barrier, regulating intestinal microecology, resisting oxidation, lowering blood sugar and blood lipid as well as improving immunity. Therefore, the common components of food and medicine lays a material foundation for their application in medical care.

2.3 Shared Source in Theory

Because of the same source of medicine and food, and the common goal is to keep people healthy, it is objectively required that they should have common theoretical guidance. The application of food and medicine is guided by the TCM theories such as the holistic view and treatment based on syndrome differentiation. They also include the theory of holism, balance, *yin* and *yang*, five-elements, nature, taste, tropism, the tendency of ascending, descending, floating and sinking, treatment individualized to patient, season and locality.

3　Items

In the *Notice on Further Regulating the Management of Health Food Raw Materials* (*Wei Fa Jian Fa* [2002] *No.* 51) issued by the former Ministry of Health in 2002, there are 86 items that are both food and medicine, including *Dingxiang* (*Caryophylli Flos*), *Bajiao Huixiang* (*Anisi Stellati Fructus*), *Daodou* (*Canavaliae Semen*), *Xiaohuixiang* (*Foeniculi Fructus*), *Xiaoji* (*Cirsii Herba*), *Shanyao* (*Dioscoreae Rhizoma*), *Shanzha* (*Crataegi Fructus*), *Machixian* (*Portulacae Herba*), *Wushaoshe* (*Zaocys*), *Wumei* (*Mume Fructus*), *Mugua* (*Chaenomelis Fructus*), *Huomaren* (*Cannabis Fructus*), *Daidai Hua* (*Flos Citri Daidai*), *Yuzhu* (*Polygonati Odorati Rhizoma*), *Gancao* (*Glycyrrhizae Radix et Rhizoma*), *Baizhi* (*Angelicae Dahuricae Radix*), *Baiguo* (*Ginkgo Semen*), *Baibaindou* (*Lablab Semen Album*), *Baibiandouhua* (*Flos Lablab Albus*), *Longan Aril* (*Longan Arillus*), *Juemingzi* (*Cassiae Semen*), *Baihe* (*Lilii Bulbus*), *Roudoukou* (*Myristicae Semen*), *Rougui* (*Cinnamomi Cortex*), *Yuganzi* (*Phyllanthi Fructus*), *Foshou* (*Citri Sarcodactylis Fructus*), *Tianxingren* (*Semen Armeniacae Dulce*), *Kuxingren* (*Armeniacae Semen Amarum*), *Shaji* (*Hippophae Fructus*), *Muli* (*Ostreae Concha*), *Qianshi* (*Euryales Semen*), *Huajiao* (*Zanthoxyli Pericarpium*), *Chixiaodou* (*Vignae Semen*), *Ejiao* (*Asini Corii Colla*), *Jinejin* (*Galli Gigerii Endothelium Corneum*), *Maiya* (*Hordei Fructus Germinatus*), *Kunbu* (*Eckloniae Thallus*), *Zao* (*Fructus Jujubae*), *Luohan Guo* (*Siraitiae Fructus*), *Yuliren* (*Pruni şemen*), *Jinyinhua* (*Lonicerae Japonicae Flos*), *Qingguo* (*Canarii Fructus*), *Yuxingcao* (*Houttuyniae Herba*), *Shengjiang* (*Zingiberis Rhizoma Recens*), *Ganjiang* (*Zingiberis Rhizoma*), *Zhizi* (*Fructus Aurantii Immaturus*), *Gouqizi* (*Lycii Fructus*), *Zhizi* (*Gardeniae Fructus*), *Sharen* (*Amomi Fructus*), *Pangdahai* (*Sterculiae Lychnophorae Semen*), *Fulin* (*Poria*), *Xiangyuan* (*Citri Fructus*), *Xiangru* (*Moslae Herba*), *Taoren* (*Persicae Semen*), *Sangye* (*Mori Folium*), *Sangshen* (*Mori Fructus*), *Juhong* (*Citri Exocarpium Rubrum*), *Jiegeng* (*Platycodonis Radix*), *Yizhiren* (*Fructus Alpinae Oxyphyllae*), *Heye* (*Nelumbinis Folium*), *Laifuzi* (*Raphani Semen*), *Lianzi* (*Nelumbinis Semen*), *Gaoliang Jiang* (*Alpiniae Officinarum Rhizoma*), *Dan Zhuye* (*Lophatheri Herba*), *Dan Douche* (*Sojae Semen Praeparatum*), *Juhua* (*Chrysanthemi Flos*), *Juju* (*Cichorii Herba*), *Huangjiezi* (*Semen Brassicae Junceae*), *Huangjing* (*Polygonati Rhizoma*), *Zisu* (*Perillae*), *Zisuzi* (*Perillae Fructus*), *Gegen* (*Puerariae Lobatae Radix*), *Heizhima* (*Sesami Semen Nigrum*), *Heihujiao* (*Fructus Piperis*), *Huaimi* (*Flos Sophorae Immaturus*), *Huaihua* (*Sophorae Flos*), *Pugongying* (*Taraxaci Herba*), *Fengmi* (*Mel*), *Feizi* (*Torreyae Semen*), *Suanzaoren* (*Ziziphi Spinosae Semen*), *Xianbaimaogen* (*Imperatae Rhizoma*),

Xianlugen（*Phragmitis Rhizoma*），*Fushe*（*Agkistrodon Halys*），*Jupi*（*Citri Reticulatae Pericarpium*），*Bohe*（*Menthae Haplocalycis Herba*），*Yiyiren*（*Coicis Semen*），*Xiebai*（*Allii Macrostemonis Bulbus*），*Fupenzi*（*Rubi Fructus*），*Huoxiang*（*Herba Agastache Rugosae*）.

In November 2014, the National Health and Famiiy planning Committee issued *Administrative Measures for the Catalogue of Substances that are Edible and Medicinal According to Tradition*（*Draft Version*）. 15 categories were added, including *Renshen*（*Ginseng Radix et Rhizoma*），*Shanyinhua*（*Lonicerae Flos*），*Yansui*（*Coriandrum sativum Linn.*），*Songhuafen*（*Pini Pollen*），*Yousong*（*Pinus Tabuliformis Carr.*），*Fenge*（*Puerariae Thomsonii Radix*），*Buzhaye*（*Microctis Folium*），*Xiakucao*（*Prunellae Spica*），*Danggui*（*Angelicae Sinensis Radix*），*Shannai*（*Kaempferiae Rhizoma*），*Xihonghua*（*Croci Stigma*），*Caoguo*（*Tsaoko Fructus*），*Jianghuang*（*Curcumae Longae Rhizoma*）*And Biba*（*Piperis Longui Fructus*）.

In November 2019, the National Health and Health Commission and the State Administration of Market Supervision jointly issued the*Notice on Piloting the Material Management of 9 Substances such as Dangshen*（*Codonopsis Radix*），*which is both food and Chinese herbal medicine according to tradition*（*Guowei Food Letter*［2019］*No.*311）. It is proposed that the production and management of *Dangshen*（*Codonopsis Radix*），*Roucongrong*（*Cistanches Herba*），*Tiepishihu*（*Dendrobii Officinalis Caulis*），*Xiyangshen*（*Panacis Quinquefolii Radix*），*Huangqi*（*Astragali Radix*），*Lingzhi*（*Ganoderma*），*Shanzhuyu*（*Corni Fructus*），*Tianma*（*Gastrodiae Rhizoma*）*And Duzhongye*（*Eucommiae Folium*）should be carried out.

第五节　养生菜肴
（Healthy Recipes）

　　菜肴，是指用肉类、蔬菜、水产品、果品等原料，经过切配和烹调加工制作成的一类食品。我国菜肴品种丰富，流派众多，制作精湛，具有选料讲究、刀工精细、配料合理、烹法多样、五味调和、工于火候、精于盛器、讲究食疗等特点。菜肴成品以色、香、味、形、器及食疗俱佳著称于世。

　　食疗食养菜肴的制作，在充分考虑营养食疗作用的基础上，还应突出菜肴的色、香、味、形，尽量做到营养疗效与色、香、味、形统一，以保证菜肴质量的完美和谐。食疗食养菜肴制作的方法以煮、炖、煨、蒸、焖、炒较好。烤、熏、煎、炸、腌等烹调方法，不利于健康，应尽量避免。

一、补益类（Recipes for Tonification）

（一）益气类

［常用食物］粳米、糯米、小米、黄豆、牛肉、鸡肉、鹌鹑、鸡蛋、土豆、胡萝卜、大枣等。

［菜肴举例］

1. 山药面（《圣济总录》）：干山药 30 克，白术 30 克，人参 5 克，面粉 500 克。将山药、白术、人参研成细粉，加入面粉、清水和面，擀切成薄片下锅煮食。可加入时令蔬菜配用。具有健脾益气功效。

2. 莲子粥（《太平圣惠方》）：莲子 25 克，糯米 50 克。将莲子去皮心研成粉，与粳米煮粥食，每日 1~2 次。具有补中益肾、聪耳明目的功效。

3. 参归炖母鸡（《乾坤生意》）：母鸡 1 只，人参 15 克，当归 15 克，葱白、生姜、黄酒、食盐各适量。母鸡去毛及内脏，冲洗干净，放入砂锅中，加清水、黄酒、葱白、生姜大火烧开，撇去污沫，改用小火炖至熟烂，再加入人参、当归、食盐，炖约 1 个小时即可。具有益气养血、益精填髓的功效。

（二）养血类

［常用食物］猪肉、羊肉、猪肝、羊肝、牛肝、甲鱼、海参、菠菜、胡萝卜、黑木耳、桑椹等。

［菜肴举例］

1. 猪肝羹（《圣惠方》）：猪肝 1 具，鸡蛋 3 个，葱白 1 根，食盐适量。猪肝洗净，去筋膜，浸泡换水数次，切成细丁，葱白切成段，以上两味原料放入豉汁中煮作羹，临熟，打入鸡蛋，待熟时即可食用。具有养血、补肝、明目的功效。

2. 桑椹龙眼膏（民间验方）：桑椹 1 000 克，龙眼 500 克，蜂蜜适量。将桑椹、龙眼洗净，放入锅内，加清水以小火煎煮至汁液黏稠时调入蜂蜜，边搅拌，边小火熬，数分钟后即可停火，待冷装瓶备用。具有养血滋阴、补肝益肾的功效。

（三）滋阴类

［常用食物］鸡蛋黄、鸭蛋黄、田鱼、乌贼、猪皮、鸭肉、桑椹、枸杞子、黑木耳、银耳等。

［菜肴举例］

1. 乌鸡羹（《太平圣惠方》）：乌骨鸡 1 只，葱白、生姜、黄酒、食盐各适量。将乌鸡宰杀后用水冲洗干净，放入锅内，加入清水煮熟，取出，去掉骨，把鸡肉切成细丁备用；生姜、葱白切成细丁备用。将鸡肉、生姜、葱白、黄酒、食盐一起上小火慢煮作羹食。具有滋补阴血的功效。

2. 清炖甲鱼（《本草备要》）：甲鱼 1 个，葱白、生姜、黄酒、食盐适量。将甲鱼杀死后，去除肠脏，然后连同山药，放入炖盅内，加水适量，隔水炖熟服用。具有滋阴清热、补虚润燥的功效。

3. 银耳羹(民间验方):干银耳 10 克,鸡蛋 1 个,冰糖适量。银耳用温水泡发,去除杂质,放入锅内,加清水,大火烧沸后转用小火,炖至银耳熟软时,加入鸡蛋、冰糖。每次 1 小碗,每日 1 次。具有补肺益肾、润燥止咳的功效。

(四)助阳类

[常用食物]羊肉、狗肉、鹿肉、兔肉、羊肾、猪肾、鸽蛋、鳝鱼、虾、淡菜、韭菜、枸杞子、刀豆、核桃仁等。

[菜肴举例]

1. 韭菜炒胡桃仁(《方脉正宗》):韭菜 200 克,胡桃仁 50 克,香油、食盐适量。胡桃仁用开水浸泡去皮,沥干备用;韭菜择洗干净,切成寸段备用。香油倒入炒锅内,烧至七成热时,加入胡桃仁,炸至金黄色,再放入韭菜、食盐,翻炒至熟。具有补肾助阳、健脑益智的功效。

2. 当归生姜羊肉汤(《金匮要略》):羊肉 500 克,当归 10 克,生姜 20 克,黄酒、食盐各适量。羊肉冲洗干净,切成小块,放入砂锅内,加黄酒、生姜、当归、清水,大火烧开,改用小火炖至羊肉熟烂,以食盐调味,分餐食用。具有温阳补虚、祛寒止痛的功效。

二、泻实类(Recipes for Purging)

(一)解表类

[常用食物]生姜、大葱、芫荽、豆豉等。

[菜肴举例]

1. 葱白芫荽汤(民间验方):大葱半根,芫荽 20 克。把大葱、芫荽洗净,大葱切成葱花,芫荽切成段备用。锅内放入清水,大火烧开,将葱花、芫荽段放入,翻滚片刻即可取下,待温饮用。具有发汗解表、宣肺通阳的功效。

2. 姜糖苏叶饮(《本草汇言》):生姜 10 克,紫苏叶 15 克,冰糖适量。先把生姜洗净切成片备用。将生姜片、紫苏叶放入茶杯中,用开水冲泡,温浸 10 ~ 15 分钟,以冰糖调味,代茶饮。或以两味原料如常法煎汤,一日 2 次。具有辛温解表、理气和胃的功效。

(二)清热类

[常用食物]苦瓜、苦菜、西瓜、绿豆、豆腐、西瓜、绿茶等。

[菜肴举例]

1. 薏苡仁绿豆粥(民间验方):薏苡仁 50 克,绿豆 50 克,粳米 100 克。将薏苡仁、绿豆、粳米洗净,放入锅中,加清水以大火烧开,再改用小火,煮至豆熟米烂即可。具有清热、解暑、化湿的功效。

2. 五汁饮(《温病条辨》):梨 1 000 克,鲜藕 500 克,鲜芦根 100 克,鲜麦冬 50 克,鲜荸荠 500 克。先把 5 种原料洗净，然后将芦根切成段，加水煎汤取汁；梨去皮核，荸荠去皮，鲜藕去节，麦冬切碎或剪碎，将处理过的后四味原料放入榨汁机内榨汁，将榨好的汁液倒入容器中，代茶饮。具有清热生津、甘寒润燥的功效。

（三）温里散寒类

［常用食物］干姜、肉桂、花椒、茴香、胡椒、辣椒、羊肉等。

［菜肴举例］

1. 胡椒煲猪肚（《饮食疗法》）：猪肚 1 个，胡椒、黄酒适量。将胡椒、食盐、黄酒入洗净的猪肚内，然后用线缝好扎紧，慢火煲煮至熟烂食用。具有健脾益胃、温中散寒的功效。

2. 川椒面（民间验方）：川椒粉（花椒）5 克，面粉 200 克，淡豆豉 10 克。川椒粉与面粉拌匀，加适量清水，做成面条。锅中放入清水，烧开后，放入面条、淡豆豉、食盐，煮熟即可。具有温中散寒的功效。

（四）行气类

［常用食物］橘皮、香橼、佛手、刀豆、玫瑰花等。

［菜肴举例］

1. 葱炒佛手丝（《食物疗法》）：佛手 2 个，葱 1 根，食盐适量。佛手洗净，切成丝；葱切丝。锅内放入少量油，烧热，放入佛手丝炒至将熟时，投入葱丝、食盐，翻炒片刻即可。具有疏肝理气、调畅气机的功效。

2. 香橼浆（《食物疗法精萃》）：鲜香橼 1 ~ 2 个，麦芽糖适量。将香橼切碎，放入带盖的碗中，加入等量的麦芽糖，隔水蒸数小时，以香橼烂为度。每服 1 匙，早晚各 1 次。具有行气开郁的功效。

（五）活血类

［常用食物］黑木耳、山楂、酒、醋等。

［菜肴举例］

1. 双耳汤（民间验方）：黑木耳 6 克，银耳 6 克，食盐适量。将黑木耳、银耳放入碗中，用温水泡发洗净，放入锅中，加清水上火煮，至熟时加入少量食盐。具有养阴活血降脂的功效。

2. 山楂饮（《简便单方》）：山楂片 15 克，冰糖适量。山楂片洗净，与冰糖一起放入茶杯中，以沸水冲泡，温浸 10 ~ 15 分钟即可饮用，代茶饮。具有活血化瘀、通络止痛的功效。

（六）止咳化痰平喘类

［常用食物］海藻、昆布、海带、紫菜、萝卜、橘络、杏仁、梨、白果、枇杷、百合等。

［菜肴举例］

1. 杏仁炖雪梨(《饮食疗法》):杏仁 10 克,雪梨 1 个,冰糖适量。将杏仁、雪梨放入盅内,隔水炖 1 个小时,以冰糖调味,食雪梨饮汤。具有清热、化痰、平喘的功效。

2. 雪羹汤(《古方选注》):海蜇 50 克,荸荠 4 枚,食盐适量。海蜇用温水洗净,切成丝备用;荸荠去皮洗净,切成片备用。将海蜇、荸荠放入锅中,加清水以大火烧开,再改用小火,继续煮 10 分钟,以食盐调味即成。具有清热化痰、润肠通便的功效。

3. 百合杏仁粥(民间验方):鲜百合 50 克(干品 15 克),杏仁 10 克,粳米 50 克,冰糖适量。先将粳米煮熟,再将杏仁(去皮尖)、百合放入,继续煮 10 分钟即可,以冰糖调味。具有润肺止咳的功效。

Dishes are food made of meat, vegetables, aquatic products, fruits and other raw materials that are prepared in particular ways such as cutting and cooking. Chinese cuisine is rich in variety from numerous schools and exquisite in production. It is particular about material selection, and focus on excellent knife skill, reasonable food matching, diverse cooking methods, harmony in five flavors, level of attainment, exquisite containers and dietotherapy. An excellent dish is perfect in terms of color, smell, taste, look, utensils and dietotherapy.

In preparing a health dish, it is important to combine its color, smell, taste and look with its nutrition and effect as a unity, ensuring the perfect harmony of dish quality. It is suggested to adopt cooking methods such as boiling, stewing, simmering, steaming, stew and stir – frying. Avoid roasting, smoking, pan-frying, deep-frying and pickling that are not conducive to health.

1　Recipes for Tonification

1.1　Invigorating *Qi*

［Common food］ Polished round – grained rice, glutinous rice, millet, soybean, beef, chicken, quail, eggs, potatoes, carrots, jujube, etc.

［Example of Dishes］

(1) Yam Noodles (from *Shengji Zonglu*):30 g dried yam, 30 g *baizhu* (*Atractylodis Macrocephalae Rhizoma*), 5 g ginseng and 500 g flour. Grind yam, *baizhu* and ginseng into fine powder, add flour and water, roll and cut it into slices, then cook in a pot. Seasonal vegetables can be added. It has the effect of invigorating spleen and *qi*.

(2) Lotus Seed Porridge (*from Taiping Shenghui Fang*):25 g lotus seeds and 50 g glutinous rice. Remove the peel and core of lotus seeds, grind them into powder, add them in the pot with glutinous rice. Cook on the stove until it becomes porridge. Eat once or twice a day. It has the effects of tonifying the middle–*jiao* and kidney, and improving hearing and eyesight.

(3) Stewed Hen with Ginseng and Angelica (from *Qiankun Shengyi*):1 hen, 15 g

ginseng, 15 g angelica, appropriate amount of scallion, ginger, yellow rice wine and salt. Remove hairs and internal organs of the hen, put in a casserole after it is cleaned, add water, yellow wine, scallion and ginger, skim off the foam after the water is boiled on a high heat, turn to low heat until cooked and rotten, then add ginseng, angelica and salt, and simmer for about one hour. It has the effects of invigorating *qi*, nourishing blood, replenishing essence and marrow.

1. 2   Nourishing Blood

[Common food] Pork, mutton, pork liver, sheep liver, beef liver, soft – shelled turtle, sea cucumber, spinach, carrot, black fungus, mulberry, etc.

[Example of Dishes]

(1) Pork Liver Congee (from *Shenghui Fang*) : 1 pork liver, 3 eggs, 1 scallion and pinch of salt. Wash the pig's liver, remove fascia, soak repeatedly with changed water, finely diced it, cut scallion into sections, boil the two with soy sauce for congee, crack raw eggs into it before cooked. It has the effects of nourishing blood, supplementing the liver and improving eyesight.

(2) Mulberry Longan Ointment (from folk remedy) : 1000 g mulberry, 500 g longan, honey. Put the washed mulberry and longan into a pot, decoct them with water over low fire. When the decoction grows thick, add honey. Stir it while boiling over low fire. Turn off the fire after a few minutes and store it in a container when it cools. It has the effects of nourishing blood and *yin*, supplementing the liver and spleen.

1. 3   Nourishing *Yin*

[Common Food] Egg yolk, duck egg yolk, soft – shelled turtle, squid, pigskin, duck meat, mulberry, medlar, black fungus, tremella, etc.

[Example of Dishes]

(1) Thick Soup of Black – bone Chicken (from *Taiping Shenghui Fang*) : 1 black – bone chicken, with proper amount of scallion, ginger, yellow wine and salt. Put the washed black–bone chicken in a pot, add water and boil until it is done. Take it out to remove bones. Dice finely the chicken as well as ginger and scallion. Boil them over low heat with yellow rice wine and salt for a thick soup. It has the effects of nourishing blood and *yin*.

(2) Stewed Soft–shelled Turtle (from *Bencao Beiyao*) : 1 soft–shelled turtle, scallion, ginger, proper amount of salt and yellow wine. Remove the intestines of the killed soft–shelled turtle, and then put it into a stewing pot together with yam, add some water. Stew it in water. It has the effects of nourishing *yin*, clearing heat, tonifying and moistening dryness.

(3) Tremella Soup (from folk remedy) : 10 g dried Tremella, 1 egg and some sugar. Having Tremella expanded by soaking it in lukewarm water, remove impurities. Put it in a pot, add water. Boil it on a high heat and turn to low fire when it is boiled. Add eggs and sugar when it is soft and well-done. 1 small bowl of it each time, once a day. It has the effects of tonifying lung and kidney, moistening dryness and relieving cough.

1.4 Supporting *Yang*

[Common Food] Mutton, dog meat, venison, rabbit meat, sheep kidney, pig kidney, pigeon eggs, eel, shrimp, mussel, garlic chives, medlar, sword bean, walnut kernel, etc.

[Example of Dishes]

(1) Stir-fried Walnut Kernel with garlic chives (from *Fangmai Zhengzong*): 200 g leek, 50 g walnut kernel, some sesame oil and salt. Soak walnut kernel in boiling water to strip off the husk, and drain them. Cut the washed garlic chives into sections. Pour sesame oil into a frying pan. When it is 70% hot, add walnut kernels and deep-fry until they turn yellow. Then add garlic chives and salt and stir-fry until cooked. It has the effects of tonifying kidney, invigorating *yang* and improving intelligence.

(2) Mutton Soup with Chinese Angelica and Ginger (from *Synopsis of Golden Chamber*): 500 g mutton, 10 g Angelica sinensis, 20 g ginger, some yellow wine and salt. Cut the washed mutton into small pieces. Stew the mutton in a casserole with yellow wine, ginger, Angelica sinensis and water. Bring to the boil over high heat. Then turn to low heat and stew until the mutton is soft and done. Add salt and serve. It has the effects of warming *yang*, tonifying, dispelling cold and relieving pain.

2 Recipes for Purging

2.1 Relieving Exterior Syndromes

[Common Food] Ginger, green onion, coriander, lobster sauce, etc.

[Example of Dishes]

(1) Soup of Green Onion and Coriander (from folk remedy): half of green onion and 20 g coriander. Wash green onions and coriander, then chop green onions and cut coriander into sections. Put them into boiled water for a while, and serve. It has the effects of producing sweating, relieving exterior syndrome, and dispersing the obstruction of lung *yang*.

(2) Drink of Ginger and Perilla Leaves (from *Bencao Huiyan*): 10 g ginger, 15 g perilla leaves and some rock sugar. Wash ginger and cut it into slices. Put the sliced ginger and perilla leaves into a cup, and add boiling water. after 10-15 minutes, add rock sugar and take it like tea. Or decoct them, take it twice a day. It has the effects of relieving exterior syndrome, regula-

ting *qi* and harmonizing stomach.

2.2　Clearing Heat

［Common Food］Bitter gourd, bitter herbs, watermelon, mung bean, tofu, watermelon, green tea, etc.

［Example of Dishes］

（1）Porridge of Coix Seed and Mung Bean（from folk remedy）：50 g coix seed, 50 g mung bean and 100 g polished round-grained rice. Put the washed coix seed, mung bean and polished round-grained rice into a pot, and add water to boil over high fire. When it is boiled, turn to low fire and cook until the beans are done and the rice is rotten. It has the effects of clearing away heat and eliminating dampness.

（2）Drink of Five Material（from *Wenbing Tiaobian* ）：1000 g pear, 500 g fresh lotus root, 100 g fresh reed rhizome, 50 g fresh *maidong*（*Ophiopogonis Radix*）and 500 g fresh water chestnut. Wash clean the five raw materials. Cut the reed roots into sections, decoct them with water to get juice. Remove the peel and core of pears, the peel of water chestnuts and joints from fresh lotus roots. Chop or cut *maidong*. Then grind the four raw materials into a juicer. Take the juice together and take it like drinking tea. It has the effects of clearing heat, promoting fluid production and moistening dryness.

2.3　Dispelling Cold by Warming the Midlle-*jiao*

［Common Food］Dried ginger, cinnamon, Sichuan pepper, fennel, pepper, chili, mutton, etc.

［Example of Dishes］

（1）Stewed Pig Stomach with Pepper（from *Diet therapy* ）：1 pig stomach, pepper and some yellow rice wine. Stuff pepper, salt and yellow wine into the washed pig stomach, then tie it up tightly with thread. Simmer it on low heat until it is thoroughly done. It has the effect of invigorating spleen and stomach, dispelling the cold by warming the middle-*jiao*.

（2）Sichuan Pepper Noodles（from folk remedy）：5 g Sichuan pepper powder（pepper）, 200 g flour and 10 g light fermented soybean. Mix Sichuan pepper powder with flour, add water, and make noodles. Put water into the pot, and bring to the boil then add noodles, light fermented soybean and salt, and cook until it is done. It has the effect of dispelling the cold by warming the middle-*jiao*.

2.4　Promoting *Qi*

［Common Food］Orange peel, citron, fingered citron, sword beans, roses, etc.

[Example of Dishes]

(1)Stir-fried Shredded Fingered Citron with Onion (from *Shiwu Liaofa*):2 fingered citron,1 onion and proper amount of salt. Cut the washed fingered citron and onion into shreds. Heat up a small amount of oil in the pan. Once hot,add shredded fingered citron and stir-fry until almost cooked. Then add shredded onion and salt,and stir-fry for a while. It has the effects of soothing liver and regulating *qi*.

(2) Citron Pulp (from *Shiwu Liaofa Jingcui*):1-2 fresh citron and proper amount of maltose. Put the chopped citron in a bowl with a lid,and add the same amount of maltose. Then steam it for several hours until citron is done. Take one spoon of it in the morning,and one at night. It has the effect of promoting *qi* circulation.

2.5　Promoting Blood Circulation

[Common Food] Black edible fungus,hawthorn,wine,vinegar,etc.

[Example of Dishes]

(1)Soup of Tremella and Black Edible Fungus (from folk remedy):6 g black edible fungus,6 g tremella and pinch of salt. Put black edible fungus and tremella into a bowl,soak them in lukewarm water,wash clean,put them into a pot,add clear water and boil,and add a small amount of salt until they are well done. It has the effects of nourishing *yin*,promoting blood circulation and reducing lipid.

(2)Drink of Hawthorn (*Jianbian Danfang*):15 g hawthorn slices and some rock sugar. Put the washed hawthorn slices and rock sugar into teacups. Steep in boiling water for 10-15 minutes and serve. It has the effects of promoting blood circulation,removing blood stasis,dredging collaterals and relieving pain.

2.6　Relieving Cough,Reducing Phlegm and Allaying Asthma

[Common Food] Seaweed, *kunbu*, kelp, laver, radish, tangerine pith, almonds, pears, ginkgo,loquat,lily,etc.

[Example of Dishes]

(1)Stewed Sydney with Almonds (from *diet therapy*):10 g almonds,1 Sydney and proper amount of rock sugar. Put almonds and Sydney into a stewing pot. Simmer it for one hour,then add rock sugar and serve. It has the effects of clearing heat as well as eliminating phlegm and dampness.

(2)Soup of Jellyfish and Water chestnuts (from *Gufang Xuanzhu*):50 g jellyfish,4 water chestnuts and proper amount of salt. Wash jellyfish with lukewarm water and cut into shreds for later use. Wash the peeled water chestnuts,and cut them into slices. Put them together into a pot, add water and bring to the boil on high heat, then turn to low fire and cook for 10 minutes, and add salt. It has the effects of clearing heat, eliminating phlegm and relaxing bowel.

(3) Lily Almond Porridge (from folk remedy): 50 g fresh lily (15g dried products), 10 g almonds, 50 g japonica rice and proper amount of rock sugar. Cook japonica rice first, then add almonds (peel and tips off) and lilies after it is done. Cook for 10 minutes, and add rock sugar. It has the effect of moistening lung and relieving cough.

第六章

中医药文化国际发展
(International Development of Traditional Chinese Medicine Culture)

文化是一个民族的根脉和灵魂,文化兴盛是国家强盛和民族复兴的重要条件。近年来,我国中医药国际化发展进入"加速跑"阶段,中医药成为深化我国与他国之间卫生合作、促进人义交流的亮丽名片,特别是中医药在抗击新型冠状病毒感染和维护人民健康中展现出的独特优势举世瞩目,为全球抗疫提供了中国经验和特色良方,国际地位快速提升。当今世界,文化越来越成为国际竞争的重要因素,加快中医药文化对外传播走向世界,不仅是展示文化自信、民族自信的重要体现,也是增强国际影响、提高国家竞争力的重要基础。

Culture is the root and soul of a nation. Cultural prosperity is an importantsign for national strength and national rejuvenation. Recently, the internationalization of Chinese medicine has entered the "accelerating" era. Chinese medicine has become a bright symbol for deepening health cooperation between China and other countries, promoting cross-cultural exchange. In particular, the unique advantages of Chinese medicine in combating the COVID-19 and maintaining people's health have attracted worldwide attention. After Chinese medicine provides China's experience and characteristic prescriptions for global epidemic resistance, its international status has rapidly improved. In today's world, culture is increasingly becoming an important factor in international competition. Accelerating the dissemination of traditional Chinese medicine culture to the world is not only an important manifestation of cultural and national confidence, but also an important foundation for enhancing international influence and national competitiveness. This article will take the Confucius Institute of Traditional Chinese Medicine as an example to elaborate on the current situation of Chinese medicine international dissemination, as well as the challenges and obstacles in the this process. It will aim to enhance the world's understanding and recognition of traditional Chinese medicine, promote the vigorous development of its international communication.

第一节　中医孔子学院
（Confucius Institute of Traditional Chinese Medicine）

习近平总书记指出,中医药学是中国古代科学的瑰宝,也是打开中华文明宝库的钥匙,希望广大中医药工作者增强民族自信,勇攀医学高峰,深入发掘中医药宝库中的精华,充分发挥中医药的独特优势,推进中医药现代化,推动中医药走向世界。多年来,孔子学院在实践中创立了中外合作办学模式,实现了合作双方共建共管、共有共享,吸引了地方、学校、企业和社会各界的广泛参与,发展为覆盖面广、包容性强的语言文化传播知名品牌。中医孔子学院更是依托中医药特色,以中医药文化教育作为汉语传播的重要载体,发挥中医药文化在凝聚中国古代哲学智慧、健康养生理念、防病治病的理法方药等方面的特色优势,更好地贴近当地民众健康需求、学习需求、职业需求,从更加实际的角度给世界民众提供一个认识和了解中华优秀传统文化的平台。

一、中医孔子学院起源（Origin of Confucius Institute of Traditional Chinese Medicine）

（一）孔子学院的成立

2004 年海外第一家孔子学院在韩国首尔成立,主要促进中韩两国之间的交流,同时传播中国博大精深的汉字文化,从而掀起了全球学中国话、写中国字的热潮。通过孔子学院,也向世界揭开了东方大国的神秘面纱,向全球展示活力的中国面貌。

孔子学院是中外合作建立的非营利性教育机构,致力于适应世界各个国家和地区人民对汉语学习的需要、对中国语言文化的了解,加强中国与世界各国教育文化的交流合作,发展中国与外国的友好关系,发展儒家文化,促进世界多元文化发展,构建和谐世界。孔子学院是一个主要进行汉语教学和中外交流培训的平台,在这里可以收纳世界各地汉语爱好者,也可以培养汉语老师,同时可以提供汉语教师资格认证证书,全面而具体地满足外国友人对中国文化的需求。

除学术交流外,孔子学院还是各国国际交流的重要场合,开展多种具有特色的交流文化活动,推动两国之间的文化融合,互相吸取精髓,切实推进汉语国际化。由于特色的办学模式以及丰富多彩的文化交流活动,孔子学院成为国际友人非常喜爱的交流场所,在这里可以更细致全面地了解真实的中国。与此同时,孔子学院也成了国外众多中国迷的权威所在,因为这里可以提供学习者最规范的汉语学习、最权威的汉语历史讲述。

目前,162 个国家和地区开办了 541 所孔子学院 1170 个孔子课堂。这样的数量之下,不仅增加了汉语文化在全球范围内的影响力,也推动了国家和国家之间的文化交流进程。

（二）中医孔子学院的成立

中医孔子学院是在孔子学院的基础上,以中医药文化的推广和对外传播为目的建立的一种非营利性教育机构,以中医学为切入点推广中国文化,旨在向广大外国受众普及中医药知识以及介绍中国文化。

中医孔子学院作为教育对外开放和中外人文交流的前沿机构,是中医药文化海外传播的有效载体之一。2007 年中国国家汉语国际推广领导小组办公室与英国伦敦南岸大学共同签署了关于合作建设伦敦中医孔子学院的协议书,黑龙江中医药大学、哈尔滨师范大学与英国伦敦南岸大学联合承办该项目。截至 2020 年底,13 个国家和地区开办了17 所中医孔子学院和孔子课堂,78 个国家 240 多所孔子学院开设了中医、太极拳等课程。

二、中医药文化传播要素(Elements of Traditional Chinese Medicine Cultural Communication)

以伦敦中医孔子学院为例,文化传播要素主要包括以下内容。

（一）汉语言教学活动

伦敦中医孔子学院提供高质量的汉语课程,并根据学生不同的情况,提供一对一的辅导和小组课程。在考试方面,开设汉语水平考试(HSK)、汉语水平口语考试(HSKK)和中小学生汉语考试(YCT)等考试服务。因与黑龙江中医药大学和哈尔滨师范大学有合作关系,学院在汉语言教学方面提供为期 2 周的中国暑期夏令营和孔子学院奖学金,鼓励学生们来到中国,更好地体验中国文化和促进中文学习。

（二）中医学课程

提供中医学课程的教学内容包括中医基础理论、针灸推拿、汉语课程、中医历史和临床实践等,以针灸为主。学院目前开设有 3 年全日制和 5 年非全日制课程。此外,学院建有 2 所临床教学门诊,为学生提供了临床实践的良好平台。学习期间,学生还要到黑龙江中医药大学实习基地参加至少 0.5 年临床实习。学生毕业后可直接获得针灸师职业资格,成为英国针灸协会的会员并开业接诊。

（三）文化活动

伦敦中医孔子学院自 2008 年正式运营以来,积极开展推广中医药文化和中国文化的各类活动,内容包括节庆活动、文化体验、中医养生、来华游学、展览巡演等。学院每年固定的文化活动有展览巡演、"中华养生周"、伦敦中小学教师代表团访华、太极免费教学和中医药文化讲座等。其品牌项目"中华养生周"活动在英国 16 个城市的 42 所中小学及高等院校举办。

（四）传播媒介

线下宣传：向英国当地政府、部门发邀请信，向小学、中学、大学及机关单位送明信片，发放海报，并联络英国其他的孔子学院协助宣传。

线上宣传：包括学院的官方网站和Twitter，并借助新闻媒体为其宣传。

（五）传播对象

英国中小学及高等院校的学生和对中医感兴趣的大众。

三、中医孔子学院的作用（Influence of the Confucius Institute of Traditional Chinese Medicine）

传播是一项必须履行一定功能的社会活动，从功能研究的角度，中医孔子学院在国际传播的过程中对当地社会和民众发挥了巨大的教育作用，对接高等教育、职业教育和社区教育，创造了一种重视教育、具有强烈教育意识的社会环境，促进民众积极吸收和学习中医药文化知识。《中国国家形象全球调查报告2018》中显示，在接触或体验过中医药文化的海外受访者中，81%对中医药文化持有好印象。中医成为海外受访者眼中最能代表中国文化的元素之一。中医孔子学院/课堂多年来致力于将中医孔子学院打造为综合文化交流平台，积极拓展渠道，发掘资源，开展多层次的学术、科研、医疗、教育、文化等活动，不断推动中医药文化在当地普及推广，提升中医药文化的国际影响力。经过多年的发展，中医孔子学院已各具规模和特色，深受当地民众欢迎。

四、中医孔子学院海外传播面临的挑战（Challenges of Confucius Institutes of Traditional Chinese Medicine in Overseas Communication）

从总量上看，中医孔子学院仅占全球孔子学院总数的2%，总体数量较少、规模较小。中医孔子学院在发展的过程中，在办学层次、医疗服务、科学研究等领域有所突破，但从整体上来看，还面临一些挑战。

（一）发展分散，协调不足

由于地域差异，中医孔子学院发展初期对所在国经济文化、医疗体系、法律法规、教育政策等情况掌握并不十分全面、深入，并受到合作方高校自身发展追求的限制，在中外合作当中存在一些普遍问题且发展规模受限。

（二）供给单一，资源不足

目前，大部分中医孔子学院由一所中方院校承办，资源供给相对单一。面对当地学生不同层次、不同类别的中医药学习需求，单一中方院校面临资源不足的挑战，如提供多语种、多层次、形式新颖、内容适用的中医药对外教材；保证持续稳定派出大量能够同时具备中医药文化国际推广和中医药专业对外教育能力的优秀师资；长期坚持推出多元化、高层次、有品牌影响力的文化活动。

（三）地域分化，整合不足

中医孔子学院需要加大与所在国的传统医学教育的发展合作，取得教育、医疗领域的专业认证，以稳固其发展基础，不断扩大其影响力。面对挑战，一是要取得其所在大学、所在国教育系统的传统医学（补充替代医学）教育学分认可；二是要取得所在国卫生/健康部门相关资格证书的考试许可，而各国、各地区认证的程序不同，具体要求也各不相同。

（四）范围较窄，影响力不足

由于文化背景和历史发展的不同，中医孔子学院所在国的卫生管理模式大部分建立在现代医学体系上，中医药面临政策和技术等方面的壁垒。传统医药在大多数国家处于补充和替代地位，辐射范围较窄。

五、中医孔子学院突破挑战的方式（Suggestions for Confucius Institutes of Traditional Chinese Medicine）

基于以上问题，有学者提出：加强统筹顶层设计，整合资源，发挥核心平台优势，解决关键问题；加快完善"一带一路"沿线国家中医孔子学院布局；充分发挥高校教育研究职能，构建多元化、开放式中医药海外教育体系；切实发挥工作联盟枢纽功能，拓展服务保障范围。

第二节　中医药文化国际传播现状
（Current International Dissemination of Traditional Chinese Medicine Culture）

文化是一个民族的根脉和灵魂，文化兴盛是国家强盛和民族复兴的重要条件。中医药文化是中华优秀传统文化的瑰宝，既涵盖了中华民族数千年认识生命、维护健康、防治疾病的思想和方法体系，又包含着中华文化的哲学智慧、核心理念、人文精神与道德规范，是解读中国传统文化的基因图谱。近年来，我国中医药国际化发展进入加速跑阶段，中医药成为深化我国与他国之间卫生合作、促进人文交流的亮丽名片。特别是中医药在抗击新型冠状病毒感染和维护人民健康中展现出的独特优势举世瞩目，为全球抗疫提供了中国经验和特色良方，国际地位快速提升。当今世界正处于百年未有之大变局，文化成为国际竞争越来越重要的因素，加快中医药文化对外传播走向世界，不仅是展示文化自信、民族自信的重要体现,也是增强国际影响、提高国家竞争力的重要基础。

一、中医药文化对外传播的政策保障(Policy Guarantee for External Propaganda of Traditional Chinese Medicine Culture)

党和政府非常重视中医药的发展与传播。新中国成立初期,国家提出了"团结中西医"的卫生工作方针,后来又提出了"西医学习中医""中西医并重"等口号。党的十八大以来,国家对中医药的发展更加重视,国务院发布《关于促进健康服务业发展的若干意见》(国发〔2013〕4 号),将"全面发展中医药医疗保健服务"列为第四项主要任务。2015 年国务院办公厅印发《中医药健康服务发展规划(2015—2020 年)》(国办发〔2015〕32 号),这是国家层面制定的首个中医药健康服务领域的专项发展规划。同年,国家旅游局和国家中医药管理局联合下发了《关于促进中医药健康旅游发展的指导意见》。2016年国务院印发《中医药发展战略规划纲要(2016—2030 年)》(国发〔2016〕15 号),首次把中医药发展上升为国家战略。2017 年 7 月 1 日,《中华人民共和国中医药法》正式施行,这从国家法律层面对中医药的发展进行了保障。2017 年,国家中医药管理局、国家发展改革委印发《中医药"一带一路"发展规划(2016—2020 年)》(国中医药国际发〔2016〕44 号),这为中医药文化的国际传播指明了方向,提供了重要的指导。国家制定的这一系列相关政策均体现了国家对中医药发展的重视程度并致力于促进中医药文化能够走出国门、走向世界,让中医药文化在文化强国建设中发挥作用。

二、中医药文化对外传播载体(Platforms for External Propaganda of Traditional Chinese Medicine Culture)

在国外建设的孔子学院、中医孔子学院或孔子课堂、中医药海外中心、海外中国文化中心是中医药文化对外传播的重要平台。世界中医药学会联合会、世界针灸学会联合会、欧洲中国传统文化联合会等世界学术团体是中医药文化国际传播的重要力量。全国高等中医药院校是培养中医药文化对外传播人才的主阵地,承担着中医药国际教育、对外交流与合作和文化传播的职能。以同仁堂、以岭药业、云南白药等为代表的中医药企业积极开拓国际市场,在海外门店推出中医药产品的同时设置中医药特色文化展示区、开办养生体验中心,积极传播中医药文化。此外,海外数百中医药协会、数万中医诊所、数十万中医药从业人员、各种名人大家的效应也构成了中医药文化对外传播不可忽视的民间力量。

三、中医药文化对外传播内容(Contents for External Propaganda of Traditional Chinese Medicine Culture)

当前中医药文化对外传播内容包含中医药基本理论,中医疗效,针灸、推拿、拔罐等中医特色技术,养生保健知识,保健产品等,但仍多以针灸、推拿为先导。中医药基本理论传播方面:《黄帝内经》《难经》《神农本草经》《伤寒杂病论》《本草纲目》等中医经典著作的英译本已翻译完成并出版;《世界卫生组织传统医学术语国际化标准》及世界中医药学会联合会制定的《中医基本名词术语国际标准》促进中医药在国际交流中形成共同语言。中医疗效对外传播方面:中医药防治新型冠状病毒感染的"三药三方"取得了举世瞩目的成绩,国内政府部门、医院、高校、媒体等机构,组织积极搭建国际抗疫学术交流平台,与世界分享中医药抗疫疗效和经验,为全球抗疫贡献中国智慧和中国方案。此外,通过举办中国国际中医药博览会、中医药文化节等活动传播中医药文化理念、中医药特色产品等。

四、中医药文化对外传播语言（Language for External Propaganda of Traditional Chinese Medicine Culture）

目前中医药国际教育和对外传播所用语言主要是英语,其他还有西班牙语、法语、意大利语、德语、日语、俄语、拉丁语等。如《本草纲目》被翻译成日、英、法、德、俄、拉丁等多种文字,广泛传播至亚洲、欧洲、美洲众多国家;世界中医药学会联合会制定的《中医基本名词术语国际标准》有中英对照、中西对照、中法对照、中意对照、中德对照。

五、中医药文化对外传播途径（Paths for External Propaganda of Traditional Chinese Medicine Culture）

长期以来,中医药文化在海外的传播途径主要包括政府间交流合作,国际组织传播,中医海外立法,院校中医药国际教育与培训,接收和培养海外中医留学生,建立海外中医孔子学院、海外中医中心、中医药合作与交流基地,开展中医药国际合作项目、国际会议、对外文化交流活动、海外医疗服务、媒体宣传报道等,初步形成了多途径的对外传播格局。此外电视媒体、报刊等传统媒介也广泛介入,如中医药文化系列电视纪录片《本草中国》译成四国语言国际版向海外发行,《中医·世界》纪录片从国内和国外视角拍摄了中医药文化在海外的传播。

六、中医药文化对外传播成效（Achievements for External Propaganda of Traditional Chinese Medicine Culture）

2010 年"中医针灸"列入人类非物质文化遗产代表作名录;2011 年《黄帝内经》《本草纲目》列入世界记忆名录;2019 年《国际疾病分类》(第十一次修订本)(ICD-11)首次列出中医药传统医学章节,建立了以中医药为基础的病证分类体系。目前中医药已传播到 196 个国家和地区,中国与 43 个国家和地区签署了中医药专门协议,已建立 41 个中医药海外中心;162 个国家和地区开办了 541 所孔子学院、1170 个孔子课堂;13 个国家和地区开办了17所中医孔子学院和孔子课堂,78个国家240多所孔子学院开设了中医、太极拳等课程,目前海外有中医药业余教学机构约1500所,每年向全球输送约3万名中医药技术人员。随着中医药深度融入"一带一路"建设,已与沿线国家合作建设50家中医药对外交流合作示范基地,ISO/TC 249已发布中医药国际标准62项。此外,近年来中医药在国际赛事中频频亮相,有效促进了中医药文化对外传播。如2016年里约奥运会上,运动员身上的火罐印记让中医拔罐悄然火遍世界;2019年在成都举办的第十八届世界警察和消防员运动会,设置了中医药服务体验馆,在赛事期间为来自世界各地的运动员提供优质的中医药服务,让他们体验中医药的神奇魅力;2022年北京冬季奥林匹克运动会主媒体中心100平方米的"中医药文化展示空间"惊艳各国媒体记者、参赛选手和来华友人。

从国内研究层面来说,近5年中医药文化国际传播、海外传播及跨文化传播的研究热度不断提升,研究范畴不断扩大,学界给予中医药文化国际传播的关注度越来越高,但海外相关研究多为中草药的资源开发与利用、中医药语言翻译问题、海外中医教学相关研究,多重视数据及中药科学性研究。总体来说,目前中医药文化国际传播既面临发展机遇,又存在诸多问题和挑战。

第三节　中医药文化国际传播面临的挑战
(The Challenges Faced by the International Dissemination of Traditional Chinese Medicine Culture)

当前中医药国际化正处于加速发展的关键时期,既面临广阔的发展前景,同时,也存在诸多亟待解决的问题。

一、中医药文化国际化传播中的问题(Issues in the International Communication of Traditional Chinese Medicine Culture)

(一)中医药文化传播国际化传播的人员专业素质不高

目前,中医药文化国际化传播的主体主要有政府机构、中医药院校、中医药医疗机构、国内外中医药从业者等。中医药文化作为中华文化的分支,其也沿袭了中华中庸文化的特点,中医药资料中的许多内容的表达较为晦涩难懂,由于中西方文化间的巨大差异,如何将国人都很难理解的古文语句翻译成大众均可明白的现代语句并传播出去成为一个难题,这就对从事中医药资料翻译工作的人员提出了非常高的要求。然而,许多翻译人员由于缺乏中医药专业知识,往往无法准确地将相关内容翻译准确;但是大多数高等中医药院校学科教育存在着专业教师有过硬的医学基本功和丰富的诊疗经验,但外语语言交际能力相对薄弱,不能胜任中医双语教学。所以,从事中医药国际化传播人员的专业素质还有待提高。

（二）中医药文化的核心价值没有得到真正的传播

中医药文化包括精神文化、行为文化和物质文化。有学者认为中医药文化核心价值至少体现在4个方面,分别为生命价值观、思想价值观、科学价值观和伦理价值观。目前国外虽然也逐渐接受中医药治疗,但是他们接受的范围也主要局限于针灸、拔罐等技术,中医药中天人合一、顺其自然、辨证施治、阴阳平衡、扶正祛邪、整体观念、三因制宜等思想并没有得到真正的传播,西方学者仍然认为这些观念缺乏证据支撑,但这些理念正是中医药文化的核心价值体现,中医药文化核心价值是中医药精神的集中体现,只有中医药文化核心价值得以传播,才能真正实现中医药文化国际化。

（三）中医药文化国际化传播的渠道较为单一

传播的载体、传播的效果也会产生重要的影响,目前中医药文化的国际化传播,主要还是通过政府在海外设立的中医中心以及公派的医务人员进行,另外还通过中医药相关书籍进行传播。但是,国外市场上的很多中医药书籍并非中国人撰写,例如英国人诺娜·弗兰格林出版的《五行针灸指南》,美国市场上也售卖着美国人自行编写的中医按摩保健类书籍。此外,国内可以看到大量的西医类的外文杂志,相反,很少有英文版的中医药类杂志发行到国外。因为传播渠道的单一化,在一定程度上也影响了中医药文化国际化传播的进程推进。

（四）中医药标准化建设发展薄弱

标准化是行业发展和获得认同的重要支柱,中医药标准化是中医药国际化发展的重要基础,但目前无论从行业标准、国家标准还是国际标准来看,中医药标准化建设亟待加强。从当前中西医发展的国际大环境来看,低标准化现状明显削弱了中医药的国际话语权,对中医药的认识错杂不一,缺乏统一共识,导致国外民众对中医药的认同度降低,阻碍了中医药文化传播。

（五）中医药文化对外传播品牌打造不足

中医药文化国际传播除了被列入世界非物质文化遗产的针灸外,尚未建立起其他具有全球影响力的中医药文化亮点品牌、具有国际知名度的中医药新媒体品牌、促进中医药文化海外传播品牌项目,同时具有国际影响的喜闻乐见的影视、动漫等中医药文化传播精品打造不足。

二、推进中医药文化国际传播策略的建议(Suggestions for Promoting the International Communication Strategy of Traditional Chinese Medicine Culture)

(一)强化中医翻译课程建设,培育高阶复合型翻译人才

现阶段,中医药国际传播亟需既懂英语又懂中医并了解中国传统文化和西方文化的复合型人才,同时这种人才还要具备语言转换能力、人际沟通能力,是一种综合性、全方位的高端翻译人才。目前中医药高端翻译人才极度缺乏,无法满足中医药国际化合作与发展的需求。对此,要充分利用高校的人才培养平台,依托高校优势、高校学术资源开设中医翻译课程,注重中医学技术性翻译的实践应用,以此培养一批多元化应用型中医翻译人才。翻译课程是每一位译者的入门必修课,课程中所学内容对翻译者的业务水平具有至关重要的作用。对于中医译者而言,除了学习翻译理论与技巧外,还要增加国际传播学和现代基础医学的理论课程,提升医学素养,培育国际视角;同时,相应地增加中医英语精品课、中国古典文化、中医文化学等特色课程,丰富教学内容,努力完善其知识结构。翻译也属于一门技能课,有了上述基础知识与理论的铺垫,还要不断加强中医药英语翻译的实践,不断提升对中医经典古籍的理解能力,如《黄帝内经》《伤寒论》等不同的国际翻译版本,了解其历史及翻译特色和不足,并实际参与到相关经典的翻译工作中,在翻译实践中不断提升翻译能力。未来在翻译实践方面,可以通过与海外中医中心、中医孔子学院等相关机构合作组建翻译实践基地,不仅可以增加更多的实践机会,还能直接服务中医药文化的国际传播,提升专业价值感和认同感。此外,双语教学也是我国中医药教育国际化的重要方法,是中医药对外传播的重要窗口,如国际针灸教学不仅开阔了学生的国际视野,也使学生对针灸学习产生了更大的兴趣。因此,应鼓励全国各大中医院校以及含中医翻译专业类的高校扩大对中医翻译专业的招生,积极投入中医药翻译人才的培养工作。目前,中医药翻译课程在中医药大学的开设度很低,今后需不断增强中医翻译的师资力量,扩大招生,培养一批具有国际视野和中医药文化底蕴的中医翻译队伍。

(二)运用反向格义法解释中医药核心价值观

格义是用我国本土固有的思想哲学概念去比附解释佛教哲学的教义,帮助僧俗大众理解佛法深义的一种方法。简言之,就是用中国本来已有的学说或经典来解释外来的思想。反向格义法则是用西方哲学的概念和理论框架来研究中国传统的哲学思想。由于中西方文化和思维方式存在着很大的差异,中医药文化中蕴含的核心价值和哲学思维,如天人合一、阴阳五行、辨证论治、气血津液学说、五运六气学说等很难直接被国外特别是西方国家所接受。我们可以借助反向格义法,运用西方哲学的概念和思维框架,用

国外民众能够理解的语句对中医药文化的核心价值进行转述,从而促进中医药文化内涵被广泛接受,实现真正意义上的中医药文化国际化传播。

(三)融入新媒体时代,赋能中医药文化国际传播

新媒体的出现改变了人们交流与获取资讯的主要方式,伴随着新媒体的不断迭代更新,5G 和人工智能时代的到来,为信息的传播提供了更为高效的可能,也为中医药的国际传播创造了新的路径。一方面,要加强新媒体传播的顶层设计,建立行之有效又符合当下国内外发展的媒体制度,加强中医药国际传播内容的把关,扩大并发挥新科技优势,打造智能化的国际传播媒体技术支撑平台。同时不断加速推进中医药领域新旧媒体融合的转型升级,实现媒体、平台和内容的互融互通,建设具有权威性的中医药传播自媒体,从传播的源头提高其信息的可信度,提高新媒体的传播力;打破固有的传播思维,依托中医药的诊疗优势,制定正确的媒体发展战略,建立新的数据驱动的手段和方法,助力政府机构,以技术为手段,数据为核心,掌握数字化时代下的中医药媒体话语权。另一方面,善于借鉴汲取海外主流新媒体平台的成功经验,将中国文化这一"高语境文化"转型成更好理解与接受的"低语境文化",将博大精深的传统文化以视听等非语言的形式呈现给受众,融合不同文化和价值观的地域差异,为海外受众提供降低"文化折扣"的跨文化解读,切实有效地促进中国文化的海外传播,为社交媒体时代中医药文化的对外传播提供参考与借鉴;建立符合中医药文化发展的国际信息交流网站,线上中外医药合作平台、中医药养生平台、远程教育平台等,逐步发展成为中医药国际化资源共享的信息与媒体资源库,并在此基础上不断拓宽互联网+中医、人工智能与中医、中医药智能化适宜技术以及中医服务大数据的传播渠道,打造自主可控的国际传播中医药新平台,从点、线、面上促进媒体效果的全面提升,如将微信公众号、微博平台、移动客户端等整合成一套完整的信息传播产业链、组合成一站式"点线面"的信息传播渠道,构建中医药文化国际传播的媒体矩阵,发挥出新媒体在当今时代文化传播中的多维度传播效能。

(四)创新中医药文化对外传播内容和形式

第一,加强中医古代文化典型案例的传播。充分发挥国医大师、全国名中医优势,运用新媒体技术和方法讲述各个历史时期中医奇迹故事,如古代名医张仲景、孙思邈、华佗中医诊疗故事,增加中医药文化传播内容、形式的丰富性和有趣性。第二,加强中医医学哲学原理的传播。运用中医取类比象方法,将中医阴阳、五行、精气、脏腑等抽象的中医概念置于西方文化背景下,借用国外读者所熟悉的人物故事原型,或将其与常见的生活场景或自然现象进行关联,以增加读者感性认识和认同。第三,加强养生保健理念文化传播。抓住人们感兴趣的饮食、健康等话题,制作中医食疗、中医养生等纪录片、短视频、微视频、微电影等,提高中医药文化影响力。第四,加强中医文化内容传播方式研究。大量的成语、故事、传说、谚语中承载着中华优秀传统文化印记,其中很多蕴含着中医药智

慧、理念、方法。要扩大中医的人文外延,用人文故事讲中医,借鉴英国 BBC 创作的《中国新年》《中国创造》《中国故事》,以幽默的英语和西方熟识的表达方式让国外听众听故事里的中医,让中医药文化不但"走出去",更要"走进去"。

Currently, the internationalization of Traditional Chinese Medicine is at a critical stage of accelerated development, which enjoys a promisingprospect, but faces many problems that should be solved urgently.

1 Issues in the International Communication of Traditional Chinese Medicine Culture

1.1 The Lack of High-Quality Talents in Disseminating Chinese Medicine Culture

At present, the main bodies of international communication of Chinese medicine culture include government agencies, Chinese. As a branch of Chinese culture, traditional Chinese medicine has the same characteristics as Chinese moderation culture. What was recorded in Chinese medicine materials are difficult to understand. Because of the huge differences between Chinese and Western cultures, it is difficult to translate the sentences of classical literary style that are difficult for Chinese people to understand into popular and readily understandable ones and spread them, which puts forward high requirements for those who are engaged in the translation of Chinese medicine materials.

However, due to the lack of professional knowledge of Chinese medicine, many translators are often unable to accurately translate related contents. And professional teachers who have excellent basic medical skills and rich experience in diagnosis and treatment in most colleges and universities of traditional Chinese medicine are less competitive in foreign language communicative competence, which becomes an impediment to bilingual teaching of traditional Chinese medicine.

Therefore, it is necessary to improve the professional knowledge and bilingual skills of personnel engaged in international communication.

1.2 Failure in Disseminating the Core Value of Traditional Chinese Medicine Culture

Traditional Chinese medicine culture includes spiritual culture, behavioral culture and material culture. Some scholars believe that the core values of TCM culture are reflected in at least four aspects, namely, life value, ideological value, scientific values and ethical values.

At present, although Traditional Chinese Medicine treatment is gradually gaining recognition of foreigners, what they accept is mainly limited to acupuncture, cupping and other techniques. The ideas of TCM have not been really spread, such as harmony between man and nature, letting nature take its course, treating based on syndrome differentiation, balancing between *yin* and *yang*, strengthening body resistance and eliminating evil, considering factors of seasons, environment and body constitution in treating diseases as well as the holistic concept. Western scholars still think that these ideas are not supported by evidence, but these ideas are the embodiment of the core value of Traditional Chinese Medicine culture that represents Chinese medicine spirit. Hence, only when the core value of TCM culture is spread, can it truly realize the internationalization of Traditional Chinese Medicine culture.

1.3 Single Channel of Internationalization of Traditional Chinese Medicine Culture

The carrier and effect of communication are also important factors. At present, the international communication of Traditional Chinese Medicine culture is mainly carried out through overseasChinese medicine centers set up by the government and public medical personnel, and also through books related to Chinese medicine.

However, many Chinese medicine books in foreign markets are not written by Chinese people, such as *Wuxing Zhenjiu Zhinan* (*The Simple Guide to Five – Elements Acupuncture*) written by Nona Franglen who is from English, and the TCM massage and health care books written by Americans are also sold in American markets.

In addition, a large number of foreign magazines related to Western medicine can be seen in China. On the contrary, few English magazines of Chinese medicine are issued abroad.

It is the simplification of communication channels that affect the progression of international communication of Chinese medicine culture to a certain extent.

1.4 Weak Development of TCM Standardization

Standardization is an important pillar for the development of an industry and the recognition it gains from public. That's why TCM standardization is an important foundation for internationalization. However, from the perspective of industry standards, national standards and international standards, the standardization of Chinese medicine needs to be strengthened urgently.

In the international environment for the development of Chinese and Western medicine, the international discourse power of Chinese medicine has been weakened obviously due to the low standardization. The incorrect and miscellaneous understanding of Traditional Chinese Medicine also leads to less recognition, which hinders the spread of TCM culture.

1.5 Insufficiency of the Brand Building of Traditional Chinese Medicine Culture

In addition to acupuncture, which is listed in the world intangible cultural heritage, we have not yet established globally influential highlight brands of Traditional Chinese Medicine culture, world-known and new media of Traditional Chinese Medicine as well as projects to promote its overseas dissemination. At the same time, popular products of TCM culture such as film, television and animation with international influence are insufficient.

2 Suggestions for Promoting the International Communication Strategy of Traditional Chinese Medicine culture

2.1 Strengthening the Construction of TCM Translation Courses and Cultivation of High-level and Compound Translators

At this stage, compound talents who know both English and Chinese medicine, as well as traditional Chinese culture and Western culture, are required in the international dissemination. At the same time, this kind of talents should be equipped with bilingual skill and interpersonal communication ability, who are comprehensive, all-round and high-end translators.

Due to the extreme shortage of high-end translators of Chinese medicine, China cannot meet the needs of international cooperation and development of Traditional Chinese Medicine.

Therefore, we should make full use of the talent training platform of colleges and universities, set up TCM translation courses relying on the advantages of colleges and universities, and value the practical application of TCM technical translation, so as to train a group of diversified and applied talents.

Translation course is a compulsory course for every translator, and the content learned in the course plays a vital role in improving the translatorl's professional skills.

It is suggested that TCM translators should not only learn the related theories and skills, but also study theoretical courses of international communication and modern basic medicine, which helps to improve medical literacy and cultivate an international perspective. At the same time, the special courses such as excellent English courses of Traditional Chinese Medicine, Chinese classical culture and culturology of TCM should be added accordingly to enrich the teaching content and strive to improve learners' knowledge structure.

Translation is also a skill course. With the above basic knowledge and theory, translators should constantly strengthen TCM English translation practice, and improve the understanding of ancient Chinese medicine classics, such as *Huangdi Neijing*, *Shanghan Lun* and other different international translation versions. It requires translators to understand their history, translation characteristics and shortcomings, and participate in the translation of related classics, constantly improving translation ability in practice.

In terms of translation practice in the future, it is suggested to work in cooperation with Overseas Chinese Medicine Centers, Confucius Institutes of Chinese Medicine and other related institutions to establish translation practice bases, which can not only increase more opportunities for practice, but also directly serve the international dissemination of TCM culture and enhance professional value and identity.

In addition, bilingual teaching is also an important method for the internationalization of Chinese medicine education in China and an important window for dissemination of Chinese medicine. For example, international acupuncture teaching not only broadens students' international vision, but also makes students more interested in acupuncture learning.

Therefore, Chinese medicine colleges and universities including Chinese medicine translation majors should be encouraged to expand the enrollment of Chinese medicine translation majors and actively participate in thetraining of Chinese medicine translation talents.

At present, few courses of TCM translation are set in universities of Chinese medicine. In the future, it is necessary to continuously strengthen teaching power, expand enrollment and train a group of TCM translation talents with international vision and deep understanding of TCM culture.

2.2 Interpreting the Core Values of Chinese Medicine by Adopting Reverse *Geyi* Method

Geyi (illuminating implication) is a method to explain the doctrine of Buddhist philosophy by using the inherent ideological and philosophical concepts in China, which can help monks and laymen understand the profound meaning of Buddhism.

In short, it is to interpret foreign ideas with existing Chinese theories or classics.

The Reverse *Geyi* method is to study Chinese traditional philosophy with the concept and theoretical framework of western philosophy.

Due to the great differences between Chinese and Western cultures and ways of thinking, the core values and philosophical thinking contained in Chinese medicine culture, such as harmony between man and nature, *yin* and *yang*, five-elements, treatment based on syndrome differentiation, the theory of *qi*, blood and body fluid, as well as the theory of five movements and six *qi*, are difficult to be directly accepted by foreign countries, especially Western countries.

Therefore, with the reverse *Geyi* method, we can paraphrase the core value of Chinese medicine culture by using the concept and thinking framework of western philosophy, and expressions that foreign people can understand, contributing to the wider acceptance of the connotation of Chinese medicine culture and realization of international dissemination of Chinese medicine culture.

2.3 Empowering the International Dissemination of TCM Culture by Integrating into the New Media

The emergence of new media has changed the main ways for people to communicate and obtain information. With the continuous update of new media, the arrival of 5G and artificial intelligence era has provided much efficiency for information dissemination and created a new path for the international dissemination of Chinese medicine.

On the one hand, it is necessary to strengthen the top-level design of new media communication, establish an effective media system that conforms to the current development at home and abroad, strengthen the control of the international communication content of Chinese medicine, expand and give full play to the advantages of new technologies, and build an intelligent technical support platform for international communication media.

At the same time, it is advised to continue to accelerate the transformation and upgrading of the integration of old and new media in the field of Chinese medicine, realize the integration of media, platforms and content, build an authoritative We Media for Chinese medicine communication, improve the credibility of its information from the source of communication, and improve the communication power of new media. It is important to change traditional mode of communication. By relying on the advantages of diagnosis and treatment of traditional Chinese medicine, it is necessary to formulate a correct media development strategy and establish new data-driven means and methods, helping government agencies to amplify the voice in traditional Chinese medicine media in the digital age with technology as the means and data as the core.

On the other hand, it is significant, by learning from the successful experience of overseas mainstream new media, to transform Chinese culture, a "high context culture", into a "low context culture" that is better understood and accepted. It helps to present profound traditional culture to audiences in non-verbal forms such as audio and visual mode, narrow the gap between regions in terms of cultures and values, which contributes to providing overseas audiences with cross-cultural interpretation to reduce "cultural discounts", effectively promoting the overseas dissemination of Chinese culture, and providing reference for the global dissemination of Chinese medicine culture in the social media era. We can also establish an international information exchange website, an online Sino-foreign medical cooperation platform, a Chinese medicine health preservation platform, a distance education platform, etc., which are in line with the development of Chinese medicine culture. These platforms gradually develop into an information and media resource library for international resource sharing of Chinese medicine. On this basis, we will continuously broaden the dissemination channels of Internet and Chinese medicine, artificial intelligence and Chinese medicine, intelligent techniques of Chinese medicine as well as big data of Chinese medicine services. By doing so, an independent and controllable new platform for international dissemination of Chinese medicine is created to promote the overall improvement of media effects from points, lines and surfaces, such as integrating WeChat official account, Weibo platform and mobile client into a complete communication industry chain, a one-stop "point-line-plane" information dissemination channel. The constructed media matrix for international dissemination of Chinese medicine culture will exert its efficiency from multiple dimensions as a new media in todayl's cultural dissemination.

2.4 Innovating the Content and Form of Global Communication of Chinese Medicine Culture

We need to give full play to the advantages of Chinese medicine masters and famous Chinese medicine practitioners in China, and tell the miracle stories of Chinese medicine in various historical periods, such as the diagnosis and treatment stories of ancient famous physicians *Zhang Zhongjing*, *Sun Simiao* and *Hua Tuo*, so as to enrich the content and form of Chinese medicine culture communication and attract people's interest, with the help of new media technologies and methods.

Second, it is suggested to focus on the dissemination of the principles of TCM philosophy.

We can adopt the analogy method of traditional Chinese medicine to put the abstract concepts of traditional Chinese medicine, such as yin and yang, five-elements, essence and qi, viscera, etc., in the western cultural background, that is, utilize the archetypes of characters' stories familiar to foreign readers, or connect with common life scenes and natural phenomena, so as to increase readers' perceptual knowledge and recognition.

Third, it is suggested to enhance the dissemination of health care concepts.

We need to grasp the topics such as diet and health that people are interested in, and make documentaries, short videos, micro videos and micro movies such as TCM dietotherapy and TCM health preservation, so as to enhance the influence of TCM culture.

Fourth, it is suggested to strengthen the research on the content and mode of TCM cultural dissemination.

There is a large number of idioms, stories, legends and proverbs bearing the imprint of excellent traditional Chinese culture, many of which contain the wisdom, ideas and methods of Chinese medicine.

It is necessary to expand the humanistic denotation of Chinese medicine and tell humanistic stories about Chinese medicine. Chinese New Year, Designed in China and The Story of China created by BBC (British Broadcasting Corporation) set a good example. What we should learn from them is to let foreign listeners accept Chinese medicine in stories with humor and familiar expressions in the West, so that Chinese medicine culture is able to "go global" and "be appreciated".

参考文献

[1]官翠玲,高山,陈阳.留学生中医药文化认同研究:以中医药院校为例[M].北京:中国社会科学山版社,2022.

[2]常玉倩."一带一路"倡议下中医药文化传播策略:以《中医文化关键词》为例[J].出版广角,2020,360(6):62-64.

[3]中医中药中国行组委会.走进中医:领略中医药文化的无穷魅力[M].北京:中国中医药出版社,2019.

[4]李致重.藏象为核心的中医体系[J].中华中医药杂志,2016,31(8):2881-2888.

[5]侯江红,吕沛宛.中医养生适宜技术操作规范(海外版)[M].郑州:中原农民出版社,2022.

[6]徐森磊,张宏如,顾一煌.艾灸温热刺激对血流量的增加作用及其相关机制探讨[J].针刺研究,2018,43(11):738-743.

[7]李晓亮.拔罐[M].北京:科学出版社,2021.

[8]徐文兵.黄帝内经四季养生法[M].北京:人民卫生出版社,2019.

[9]姚新,宋阳.中医养生与食疗(中医特色)[M].3版.北京:人民卫生出版社,2022.

[10]谢果珍,唐雪阳,梁雪娟,等.药食同源的源流内涵及定义[J].中国现代中药,2020,22(9):1423-1427.

[11]逄增玉,包学菊.孔子学院与中国文化国际传播研究[M].北京:中国传媒大学出版社,2022.

[12]宁继鸣.孔子学院研究年度报告(2019)[M].北京:商务印书馆,2019.

[13]毛嘉陵,李瑞锋,侯胜田,等.中医文化蓝皮书:中国中医药发展报告(2021)[M].北京:社会科学文献出版社,2022.